Testosterone Therapy

Why You Should Not Do It

SOUTHERLAND | COPYRIGHT 2024

Contents

Introduction

As you begin this book, let's be clear about one thing: this is not your run-of-the-mill medical guide, tiptoeing around the sensitive subject of testosterone therapy. No, this is a brazen dive into the heart of a medical controversy, a realm where science meets sensationalism, and where the promise of vitality often clouds the judgment of both patients and practitioners.

This book is about unearthing the raw, unvarnished truth of testosterone therapy. We're going to strip away the glossy veneer that's been polished by aggressive marketing and media hype. Here, we're not afraid to ask hard questions or face uncomfortable truths. Why? Because when it comes to meddling with the body's hormonal balance, the stakes are sky-high.

Let's start by setting the stage. Testosterone therapy, at its core, is about introducing synthetic testosterone into the body, typically to counteract the effects of declining natural testosterone levels. Sounds straightforward, right? But scratch beneath the surface, and you'll find a labyrinth of implications, both medical and ethical.

Our thesis is simple yet provocative: testosterone therapy, as it's commonly pursued today, is often a misguided choice, fraught with potential harms and misconceptions. We're not here to deny the therapy's benefits for those who truly need it. Instead, we're here to challenge the status quo, to question whether the current trend of testosterone use is more driven by myth than medical necessity.

As you embark on this journey with us, be prepared to confront some uncomfortable realities. You'll learn about the history of testosterone use - a history that's as much about human ambition and desire as it is about medical progress. You'll delve into the biological role of testosterone, understanding how it shapes our bodies and behaviors, and why tampering with it can be like playing with fire.

The heart of our exploration will take us through the maze of media and marketing influence - a landscape where facts often become entangled with fiction, and where the health of individuals can become secondary to profits. We'll dissect the short-term side effects and the long-term health risks, backed by case studies and scientific research.

But this book is more than just a critique; it's a call to action. We'll explore the ethical and societal implications of testosterone therapy, challenging both healthcare providers and patients to think critically about its use. And finally, we'll look ahead, examining the future of hormone therapy and advocating for a more informed, cautious approach.

So, buckle up. This journey won't always be comfortable, but it's necessary. It's time to peel back the layers of testosterone therapy and look it squarely in the eye. Let's begin.

Overview of Testosterone Therapy

Testosterone therapy, often hailed as a fountain of youth, is more than just a medical treatment; it's a symbol of our relentless pursuit of vitality, strength, and sexual prowess. At its core, testosterone therapy involves the introduction of synthetic testosterone into the body, typically to combat the natural decline of this hormone in men as they age. It's like adding fuel to a dwindling fire, hoping to rekindle the flames of youth. But this isn't just a simple matter of topping up a hormone; it's a complex intervention with profound implications.

The common uses of testosterone therapy are as varied as they are controversial. For some men, it's a legitimate treatment for medical conditions like hypogonadism, where the body fails to produce enough testosterone on its own. Here, therapy is not just beneficial; it's essential. However, the plot thickens when testosterone therapy is used for non-medical reasons. We're talking about men chasing the dream of eternal youth, seeking to boost libido, increase muscle mass, improve mood, and enhance overall energy levels. This is where testosterone therapy morphs from a medical intervention into a lifestyle choice, a tool in the quest for an idealized image of masculinity.

But let's not forget, testosterone therapy isn't exclusive to men. Women, too, sometimes turn to this treatment, albeit for different reasons. In women, testosterone therapy is often used to address specific medical concerns like low sex drive or certain aspects of postmenopausal care. This use, while less common, underscores the hormone's complex role in both male and female physiology.

At this juncture, it's crucial to underscore that testosterone therapy is not a one-size-fits-all solution. While it can be life-changing for some, it's an ill-advised gamble for others. This dichotomy is the essence of the therapy's use - a balancing act between medical necessity and elective enhancement. As we delve deeper into the subsequent chapters, we'll unravel the layers of this complex and often misunderstood therapy, challenging assumptions and shedding light on the multifaceted role of testosterone in our bodies and our society.

Early Discoveries and Uses of Testosterone

The story of testosterone is a tale as old as time, or at least as old as the early 20th century, when science first began to unravel the mysteries of this potent hormone. The discovery of testosterone was not a eureka moment, but rather a series of incremental steps that gradually illuminated its crucial role in the human body. It's a narrative marked by curiosity, ambition, and, frankly, a fair share of stumbling in the dark.

Our journey into the annals of testosterone history takes us back to the 1800s, when scientists first began to suspect that testicles played a key role in male development. But it wasn't until the 1930s that testosterone made its grand entrance into the medical world. Credit for its discovery is often given to a trio of chemists: Ruzicka, Butenandt, and Hanisch, who independently synthesized the hormone. This was no small feat; it was like finding the golden key to a lock that had puzzled scientists for decades.

Once testosterone was isolated and identified, the race was on to explore its potential uses. The initial focus was largely on treating men with hypogonadism. Testosterone therapy, in these early days, was like a miracle for those who lacked natural hormone production. It was the dawn of a new era in medicine, one where a deficiency once considered untreatable was now manageable.

But, as is often the case with new medical discoveries, excitement quickly gave way to experimentation. By the 1940s and 1950s, testosterone was being touted as a cure-all for a range of conditions, from depression to impotence, from enhancing male vitality to delaying the effects of aging. It was as if doctors had stumbled upon a medical fountain of youth, and they were eager to see just how far the waters could flow.

However, this early period of testosterone use was marked by a lack of understanding and oversight. The long-term effects were not yet known, and the hormone was often administered without much thought to the potential consequences. It was a wild west of hormone therapy, a time of medical pioneers and patients who were all too often unwitting participants in a grand medical experiment.

In these early uses and discoveries, we see the seeds of today's attitudes towards testosterone therapy. The allure of a simple solution to complex problems, the seduction of the promise of eternal youth, and the underestimation of the risks involved. As we move forward into the history of testosterone, it becomes clear that while our understanding of the hormone has evolved, our fascination with its potential remains as strong as ever.

Evolution of Testosterone Therapy

The evolution of testosterone therapy in medical practices is a story that mirrors the broader trajectory of modern medicine, marked by both groundbreaking advances and cautionary tales. From its inception as a groundbreaking treatment for specific medical conditions to its current status as a highly debated intervention, testosterone therapy has undergone a significant transformation, reflecting our evolving understanding of endocrinology, patient care, and ethical medical practice.

In the early days, following its discovery and synthesis, testosterone therapy was like a new frontier in medicine, primarily used to treat men suffering from hypogonadism. This was a groundbreaking development, offering relief and a semblance of normalcy to those who had no other recourse. However, the initial euphoria and novelty soon gave way to broader applications, some of which ventured far beyond the therapy's original intent. By the mid-20th century, testosterone began to be seen not just as a treatment for deficiency, but as a tool to enhance strength, vitality, and masculinity. This period marked the beginning of testosterone's journey from a strictly medical solution to a lifestyle drug.

As we moved into the latter half of the 20th century, the medical community began to gain a deeper understanding of the hormone's role and the implications of its supplementation. This was a time of burgeoning scientific inquiry, where the effects of long-term testosterone use started to become clearer. The initial enthusiasm was tempered by emerging data about potential side effects and health risks, leading to more cautious and judicious use in medical practices. The shift was gradual, from seeing testosterone as a cure-all to understanding it as a powerful hormone with significant effects on the body's complex system.

The turn of the century brought with it a renewed interest in testosterone therapy, spurred on by advances in pharmaceutical technology and a growing focus on anti-aging treatments. Testosterone therapy began to be marketed aggressively to middle-aged and older men, often capitalizing on fears of aging and loss of masculinity. This era saw the rise of 'Low T' clinics and a surge in prescriptions, a trend that raised concerns among many in the medical community about overprescription and the trivialization of hormone therapy.

Today, testosterone therapy stands at a crossroads, caught between its proven benefits for certain medical conditions and the risks and ethical questions surrounding its use for lifestyle purposes. The medical community now approaches testosterone therapy with a more nuanced understanding, advocating for a personalized, evidence-based approach. This evolution reflects a broader shift in medicine, where patient welfare and informed decision-making are paramount, and where the allure of quick fixes is weighed against the need for thorough understanding and caution.

Current Trends in Testosterone Prescriptions

The landscape of testosterone prescriptions today is as complex and nuanced as the hormone itself. Current trends reflect a society increasingly focused on wellness and longevity, yet also reveal the pitfalls of overmedicalization and the influence of pharmaceutical marketing. Testosterone, once a niche treatment for specific medical conditions, has now entered the mainstream, riding the wave of a societal obsession with youth, vitality, and performance.

In recent years, we've witnessed a significant uptick in testosterone prescriptions, a trend driven largely by the aging population and the commercialization of male aging. Men in their middle years, confronted with the natural decline in testosterone that comes with age, are turning to hormone therapy in droves, seeking to recapture the vigor of their youth. This phenomenon has been fueled by the relentless marketing of testosterone products, which often frame normal aging as a medical condition in need of treatment. Terms like "Low T" have entered the common lexicon, emblematic of how a natural biological process has been pathologized.

The rise of specialized "Low T" clinics has further propelled this trend, offering easy access to hormone therapy, often with minimal oversight or comprehensive evaluation. These clinics, sometimes more focused on profit than patient care, have contributed to a surge in prescriptions, raising concerns about the appropriateness and safety of such widespread use. It's a classic case of supply creating its own demand, where the availability and marketing of testosterone therapy make it an attractive option for those who might not need it.

However, this increase in prescriptions has not gone unchallenged. The medical community has raised alarms about the potential overuse and misuse of testosterone therapy. There's growing concern that many men receiving therapy may not have a clear medical indication for it, and that the risks - including cardiovascular issues, prostate health concerns, and other side effects - might outweigh the benefits for these individuals. This has led to a push for more stringent guidelines and a reevaluation of prescribing practices.

Another notable trend is the increasing scrutiny and regulation of testosterone products by regulatory bodies like the FDA. Recent years have seen more stringent labeling requirements and recommendations for more careful patient screening and monitoring. These regulatory changes aim to ensure that testosterone therapy is used appropriately and safely, reserving it for cases where it is genuinely indicated.

Amidst these trends, there's also a growing call for a more holistic approach to managing symptoms associated with low testosterone. This includes a greater emphasis on lifestyle modifications, like diet and exercise, and a more critical examination of the role of testosterone supplements in overall health. It's a move towards a more balanced, less interventionist approach, where the decision to prescribe testosterone is made with careful consideration of the individual patient's circumstances and needs.

The current trends in testosterone prescriptions are a reflection of a society grappling with the complexities of aging, the allure of quick fixes, and the challenges of responsible medical practice. As we continue to navigate this terrain, the key will be finding a balance between providing legitimate medical treatment to those who need it and avoiding unnecessary and potentially harmful interventions for those who do not.

Role of Testosterone in Males and Females

Testosterone, often pegged as the quintessential male hormone, plays a starring role in the biological opera not just of men, but also of women, albeit in a more understated capacity. Its influence stretches across a spectrum of bodily functions, from the blatantly obvious to the subtly profound. In males, testosterone is like the conductor of the orchestra of masculinity, directing the development of male sexual characteristics during puberty, fueling sexual drive, and playing a critical role in sperm production. It's the hormone that deepens voices, boosts muscle mass, and carpets chests with hair. But its role isn't just skin-deep. Testosterone also contributes to bone density, red blood cell production, and overall mood and energy levels. It's a hormone that, in many ways, defines what it means to be male in a biological sense.

In females, testosterone is more of a supporting actor, present in much smaller quantities, but no less vital. It's produced in the ovaries and adrenal glands and plays a crucial role in bone strength, brain function, and the development of lean muscle mass. Testosterone in women also influences libido, menstrual health, and even fertility. Its levels fluctuate throughout a woman's life, affecting her physical and emotional well-being in ways that are only beginning to be fully understood.

However, the role of testosterone goes beyond these physical attributes. It's a hormone deeply intertwined with our overall health and well-being. In men, for instance, low levels of testosterone have been linked to a host of health issues, from obesity to heart problems to mood disorders. This has led to the view of testosterone as a kind of elixir of health, a perception that partly fuels the enthusiasm for testosterone therapy.

In women, the interplay of testosterone is equally complex. While it's a lesser-known player in female physiology, its impact is significant. Imbalances in testosterone levels in women can lead to conditions like polycystic ovary syndrome (PCOS), characterized by excess testosterone, or the loss of libido and other health issues when levels are too low.

Yet, for all its importance, testosterone is a hormone that demands a delicate balance. Too much or too little can tip the scales in either direction, leading to a range of health issues. In men, excessive testosterone can lead to aggression, acne, and even heart problems, while in women, it can cause masculinizing effects and menstrual irregularities.

Natural Fluctuations of Testosterone Levels

In the grand ballet of human biology, testosterone levels don't dance to a static rhythm; they fluctuate, ebbing and flowing in a natural cadence that reflects the complexities of our bodies. These fluctuations are not mere quirks of biology; they are fundamental to our physical and emotional well-being, playing out in a myriad of subtle yet significant ways.

For men, testosterone levels are at their peak in the morning, a fact that's not just a trivial piece of trivia but a reflection of the hormone's deep ties to circadian rhythms. But it's not just daily fluctuations that matter. Over the course of a lifetime, testosterone levels in men follow a more poignant trajectory. From the surge that triggers the wonders of puberty, these levels reach their zenith in early adulthood, only to begin a gradual, inexorable decline as men age. This natural decline, often starting as early as the 30s, is like the slow dimming of a light. It's not a dramatic drop, but a gentle descent that can, over decades, significantly impact everything from muscle mass and bone density to libido and mood.

The implications of these natural fluctuations are profound. In the realm of sexual health, for instance, the waning of testosterone can lead to a decrease in libido, erectile dysfunction, and fertility issues. But the effects are broader, potentially influencing body composition, energy levels, and even mental health. Conditions like depression and anxiety have been linked to low testosterone levels, painting a picture of a hormone that's as much about the mind as it is about the body.

In women, the dance of testosterone is more subtle but no less significant. While their bodies produce much less of the hormone, its fluctuations can still impact their health in noticeable ways. For instance, during the menstrual cycle, testosterone levels peak around ovulation, contributing to an increase in sexual desire. Similarly, as women approach menopause, the decline in estrogen is accompanied by a relative increase in testosterone, a shift that can manifest in various physical and emotional changes.

However, it's not just age that affects testosterone levels. Factors like stress, sleep, diet, and physical activity all play their part in this hormonal symphony. Chronic stress, for instance, can lead to elevated levels of cortisol, a hormone that, in excess, can suppress testosterone production. Poor sleep and an unhealthy diet can similarly take a toll, underscoring the hormone's sensitivity to lifestyle factors.

The natural fluctuations of testosterone levels, and their wide-ranging implications, highlight the hormone's central role in our health. They also underscore the importance of approaching testosterone therapy with caution. In seeking to alter these natural levels, particularly in the absence of a clear medical need, we risk disrupting a delicate balance that has both subtle and profound effects on our bodies and minds. It's a reminder that in our quest to optimize our health, respect for the body's natural rhythms is key.

Misconceptions About the Benefits

In the realm of testosterone therapy, there exists a chasm between perception and reality, a gap filled with misconceptions and half-truths about the benefits of artificially elevated testosterone levels. These misconceptions are not just harmless myths; they are potent narratives that drive individuals towards unnecessary and potentially risky treatments, buoyed by the false promise of a panacea for aging and lost vitality.

One of the most pervasive misconceptions is the idea that boosting testosterone is a shortcut to eternal youth. This modern-day fountain of youth narrative is compelling, seductive even. It plays on our deepest fears of aging and our societal obsession with youth and vigor. The promise is that with just a simple injection or gel, men can reclaim the energy, muscle mass, and libido of their younger selves. However, the reality is far more complex. While testosterone therapy can indeed alleviate symptoms of testosterone deficiency, its efficacy as an anti-aging elixir is grossly overstated. The improvements in energy, libido, and physical strength are often modest and not guaranteed. More importantly, these potential benefits come with the risk of significant side effects, a fact often glossed over in the enthusiastic marketing of testosterone products.

Another common misconception revolves around the idea that more testosterone equals more masculinity. This equation of hormone levels with manliness not only oversimplifies the complex nature of gender and identity but also ignores the fact that the body's hormonal balance is a finely tuned system. Excess testosterone can disrupt this balance, leading to a range of issues from acne and hair loss to more serious concerns like heart problems and prostate enlargement. This distortion of masculinity into a numerical hormone level is not just scientifically flawed; it's a narrative that can lead men down a path of unnecessary and risky medical interventions.

The belief in testosterone as a cure-all for a range of ailments, from depression to obesity, is another misconception with little scientific backing. While it's true that testosterone plays a role in mood, metabolism, and overall well-being, the idea that boosting testosterone is a straightforward solution to these complex health issues is misguided. Many factors contribute to conditions like depression and obesity, and oversimplifying these to a hormone deficiency does a disservice to the multifaceted nature of health and disease.

There's the misconception about the safety of long-term testosterone therapy. The narrative here is often one of reassurance, suggesting that testosterone therapy is a low-risk intervention. However, the long-term effects of artificially elevated testosterone levels are not yet fully understood. Concerns about cardiovascular health, prostate cancer, and other potential risks are still being explored, making the safety profile of long-term testosterone therapy a subject of ongoing research.

How the Media Portrays Testosterone Therapy

The media's portrayal of testosterone therapy is a masterclass in seduction and oversimplification, painting a picture that often blurs the lines between medical treatment and lifestyle choice. This portrayal is not merely a reflection of media tendencies but a powerful force that shapes public perception and influences personal health decisions. The narrative spun by the media is one of transformation and rejuvenation, a siren song that plays on deep-seated fears of aging and obsolescence.

Television commercials, magazine ads, and online articles frequently depict testosterone therapy as the gateway to renewed vigor and masculinity. These portrayals are replete with images of muscular, energetic men, living life to the fullest, implying that testosterone therapy is the secret ingredient to achieving this idealized state. The messaging is slick and compelling, often glossing over the complexities and potential risks in favor of a simple, appealing story: low testosterone is a problem, and therapy is the solution.

This narrative is further amplified by celebrity endorsements and personal testimonials, lending an air of credibility and relatability to the therapy. Celebrities and athletes, revered for their physical prowess and vitality, tout the benefits of testosterone therapy, often downplaying the medical implications in favor of personal anecdotes of transformation. These stories, while compelling, create a skewed perception of the therapy, presenting it as a lifestyle choice rather than a medical treatment with specific indications and potential risks.

Moreover, the media often fails to provide a balanced view of the scientific debate surrounding testosterone therapy. The coverage tends to be binary, either touting the miraculous benefits of the therapy or decrying it as dangerous and ineffective, with little room for nuance. This polarized reporting makes it difficult for the public to understand the true nature of the therapy, the conditions it is meant to treat, and the potential risks involved.

The role of the media in promoting the idea that natural aging processes, such as the decline in testosterone, need to be medically managed, is also significant. This narrative plays into societal fears of aging, positioning testosterone therapy as a necessary intervention to maintain youth and vitality. Such a portrayal not only misrepresents the natural aging process but also contributes to the overmedicalization of aging, turning a natural biological phenomenon into a condition that requires treatment.

In summary, the media's portrayal of testosterone therapy is a complex interplay of marketing, storytelling, and societal norms. It is a portrayal that often prioritizes appeal over accuracy, simplicity over complexity, and rejuvenation over reality. This portrayal has a profound impact on public perception and healthcare decisions, underscoring the need for more balanced, nuanced, and informative media coverage that respects the intricacies of hormone therapy and the realities of aging.

Pharmaceutical Marketing

The role of pharmaceutical marketing in promoting testosterone therapy is akin to a juggernaut driving the narrative around this medical intervention, shaping public perception, and influencing prescribing practices. This marketing is not just about promoting a product; it's about constructing a narrative, one that often prioritizes profit over patient welfare and bends the arc of medical practice towards overuse and misapplication.

Pharmaceutical companies, armed with hefty marketing budgets, deploy a wide array of tactics to push testosterone products. Direct-to-consumer advertising is a key strategy, with commercials and print ads portraying testosterone therapy as a panacea for a range of age-related concerns. These ads skillfully weave a tale of lost masculinity and waning vitality, only to present testosterone therapy as the hero of the story, the solution to reclaiming a youthful, energetic life. The messaging is relentless and pervasive, infiltrating every corner of media from TV screens to web banners.

But the marketing machine doesn't stop at direct-to-consumer efforts. Physicians are also a primary target, with pharmaceutical reps providing doctors with product information, free samples, and sometimes, incentives to encourage prescriptions. These practices, while not inherently unethical, can create conflicts of interest and skew prescribing practices. The line between educating healthcare providers and incentivizing them to prescribe a particular product becomes blurred, raising questions about the impartiality of medical decision-making.

The pharmaceutical industry's influence extends to the framing of low testosterone as a widespread medical problem in need of treatment. By funding studies and promoting the concept of "Low T," these companies have been instrumental in medicalizing a natural part of aging. The result is an expansion of the market for testosterone products, tapping into a demographic that extends far beyond those with clinically significant hormone deficiencies.

Furthermore, the marketing often downplays the potential risks and side effects of testosterone therapy, presenting it as a low-risk intervention. The emphasis is on the benefits, with less attention paid to the therapy's long-term implications, the nuances of patient suitability, or the importance of careful monitoring. This skewed portrayal can lead to unrealistic expectations and underappreciation of the therapy's risks among both patients and healthcare providers.

Pharmaceutical marketing plays a central role in driving the popularity of testosterone therapy, shaping how it is perceived and utilized in society. This influence raises critical questions about the balance between commercial interests and patient health, the integrity of medical practice, and the need for more stringent regulation of pharmaceutical marketing. As we navigate the complex landscape of hormone therapy, understanding the impact of this marketing is crucial in ensuring that medical decisions are made based on patient welfare, not market influence.

Misleading or Exaggerated Advertising

Diving into the world of testosterone therapy, we encounter a landscape littered with case studies of misleading or exaggerated advertising campaigns, each one a testament to the power of marketing to shape public perception and influence healthcare decisions. These campaigns, often more focused on selling a narrative than presenting facts, have played a significant role in the overuse and misunderstanding of testosterone therapy.

One such case involved a major pharmaceutical company that aggressively marketed a testosterone product as a remedy for a fabricated condition they dubbed "Low T". This term, catchy and clever, was plastered across TV ads, billboards, and magazine spreads, presenting common signs of aging like fatigue and decreased libido as symptoms of a widespread medical issue. The campaign was wildly successful, leading to a surge in prescriptions. However, it was later criticized for trivializing the medical use of testosterone and contributing to its overprescription. The FDA eventually stepped in, reprimanding the company for overstating the benefits and downplaying the risks of therapy, a move that highlighted the often blurred line between marketing and medical advice.

Another case study involves a testosterone gel product that was marketed as a lifestyle drug for men facing the natural decline of testosterone with age. The ad campaign featured images of robust, energetic men, implying that the gel could restore vitality and reverse the effects of aging. This portrayal played into societal insecurities about aging and masculinity, effectively turning a hormone therapy into a must-have lifestyle product. However, the ads failed to adequately disclose the potential risks, including the transfer of testosterone to women and children through skin contact. The company faced legal consequences for these misleading practices, underscoring the ethical and legal pitfalls of such aggressive marketing.

A third example comes from an online marketing campaign, where a testosterone supplement was touted as a natural alternative to prescription therapy. The campaign used pseudo-scientific jargon and misleading testimonials to promote the product, claiming it could boost testosterone levels without the side effects of traditional therapy. This claim was later debunked, and the company was fined for false advertising. The case highlighted the dangers of misinformation in the largely unregulated supplement market, where the line between truth and marketing is often dangerously thin.

These case studies are not just isolated incidents; they reflect a broader trend in the marketing of testosterone therapy and supplements. They reveal how easily medical treatments can be commodified and how public health can be compromised in the pursuit of profit.

They also underscore the need for more stringent regulation of pharmaceutical and supplement marketing, to ensure that the information reaching the public is accurate, balanced, and in the best interest of patient health. As we continue to grapple with the implications of testosterone therapy, these case studies serve as cautionary tales, reminding us of the importance of critical thinking and informed decision-making in the face of persuasive marketing.

Psychological Impacts

The psychological landscape altered by testosterone therapy in the short term is as tumultuous as a stormy sea. It's a realm where mood swings and aggression can surge like unexpected waves, catching both the individual and their loved ones off guard. The impact of testosterone on mental health is a narrative often overshadowed by its physical effects, yet it's a story that demands to be told, for the mind is as vulnerable to the whims of this hormone as the body.

The introduction of testosterone therapy can be akin to throwing a switch in the brain. Some individuals report dramatic mood swings, oscillating between highs and lows with a volatility that can be both bewildering and distressing. It's as if the therapy stirs a pot of emotional unrest, bringing to the surface feelings that are intense and often difficult to manage. This rollercoaster of emotions isn't just hard on the individual; it can strain relationships and disrupt daily life.

Aggression, too, can rear its head, an unwelcome guest in the psychological house that testosterone therapy builds. This increase in aggression isn't just a stereotype; it's a real and often disconcerting side effect for some. The heightened aggression can manifest in irritability, impatience, or even anger outbursts, turning the dial up on emotions that were once more easily controlled. It's as if testosterone therapy amplifies certain emotional responses, leaving individuals feeling like they're at the mercy of their own heightened reactions.

Beyond mood swings and aggression, other mental health concerns can also surface. Anxiety and depression, those twin specters of mental unrest, have been reported as side effects of testosterone therapy. It's a paradoxical twist, where a treatment sought for well-being becomes a trigger for mental health challenges. These issues are not just passing clouds; they can cast long shadows, affecting quality of life and overall well-being.

It's important to note that these psychological impacts are not universal; they don't strike everyone with the same intensity. But their potential presence is a crucial consideration for anyone contemplating testosterone therapy. Mental health, often more elusive and complex than physical health, requires careful monitoring during therapy.

The short-term psychological impacts of testosterone therapy — mood swings, aggression, and other mental health concerns — are vital pieces of the puzzle. They remind us that testosterone's influence extends beyond muscle mass and libido, reaching into the intricate workings of the mind. As we navigate the choppy waters of hormone therapy, a clear understanding and vigilant monitoring of these psychological effects are essential, ensuring that the quest for physical health does not come at the cost of mental well-being.

Cardiovascular Risks

Steroids, often viewed through the lens of their muscle-building prowess, cast a much darker shadow when it comes to their impact on the cardiovascular system. This intricate and vital network, the lifeblood of our very existence, is subjected to a barrage of harmful effects when anabolic steroids enter the bloodstream. To fully grasp the gravity of this issue, one must dive deep into the physiological changes and repercussions that these substances inflict upon the cardiovascular system.

At the heart of the matter, quite literally, is the heart itself. Anabolic steroids, synthetic variations of the male sex hormone testosterone, are known to induce hypertrophy – an increase in muscle size. While this might sound beneficial for skeletal muscles, it's a detrimental phenomenon for the heart. The heart, a muscular organ, responds to steroids in a similar fashion, undergoing hypertrophy, particularly in the left ventricle, the chamber responsible for pumping oxygen-rich blood throughout the body. This thickening of the heart's walls may sound innocuous or even beneficial at first, but it is far from it. The increased mass in the heart's muscular wall can lead to a decrease in its efficiency and flexibility. A heart that is less flexible and efficient struggles to pump blood effectively, which can lead to a host of problems, including a reduced capacity to exercise, shortness of breath, and in severe cases, heart failure.

Delving deeper into the vascular system, steroids enact a sinister play on cholesterol levels. Cholesterol, often vilified, is essential for various bodily functions, including the production of hormones and vitamin D. However, balance is key, and steroids disrupt this balance severely. They increase Low-Density Lipoprotein (LDL) cholesterol, the so-called 'bad' cholesterol, while decreasing High-Density Lipoprotein (HDL) cholesterol, the 'good' cholesterol. This shift fosters the build-up of plaques inside the arteries, a condition known as atherosclerosis. These plaques narrow the arteries, reducing blood flow and increasing the risk of heart attack and stroke.

Moreover, anabolic steroids can lead to an increase in blood pressure. This rise in blood pressure is a silent yet formidable foe, often going unnoticed until significant damage is done. Elevated blood pressure strains the heart, forcing it to work harder to pump blood. Over time, this relentless pressure can weaken the heart, contributing to heart disease and increasing the risk of heart failure.

In addition to these effects, steroids also influence blood clotting factors, tilting the scales toward a hypercoagulable state. This means the blood becomes more prone to clotting, which is particularly dangerous when coupled with the plaque build-up in the arteries. The formation of a clot inside a narrowed artery can lead to catastrophic events like a heart attack or stroke, as the clot can completely block the flow of blood to vital organs.

Beyond these direct effects on the heart and blood vessels, steroids also impact other factors that indirectly contribute to cardiovascular disease. They can lead to an increase in body weight and body mass index (BMI), often through an increase in muscle mass and water retention. While increased muscle mass might be the desired effect for some users, the additional weight still requires the heart to work harder, exacerbating any existing cardiovascular issues. Additionally, steroids can lead to insulin resistance and changes in glucose metabolism, factors that contribute to the development of diabetes – another risk factor for heart disease.

The confluence of these factors – hypertrophy of the heart, atherosclerosis, high blood pressure, hypercoagulability, and metabolic changes – creates a perfect storm for cardiovascular disease in steroid users. It's a silent epidemic, often overshadowed by the more visible muscle growth and performance enhancements. Yet, the real battle is waged deep within, in the arteries and the heart, often unnoticed until it's too late.

Hormonal Imbalance

The long-term health risks associated with hormonal imbalances, particularly due to prolonged testosterone supplementation, are a topic of growing concern and significance in the realm of medical science. Testosterone, a hormone primarily associated with male sexual development and function, also plays a vital role in various bodily systems. Its supplementation, often sought for its perceived benefits like increased muscle mass, improved sexual function, and enhanced overall vitality, can have far-reaching and detrimental effects when used in excess or for prolonged periods.

At the forefront of these risks is the disruption of the body's natural hormonal balance. The endocrine system, a delicately balanced network, is highly sensitive to changes in hormone levels. When exogenous testosterone is introduced into the system, the body's natural feedback mechanisms, which regulate hormone production, are disrupted. The body senses the high levels of testosterone and responds by reducing its own production of the hormone. This reduction can lead to a decrease in the production of other hormones as well, like luteinizing hormone (LH) and follicle-stimulating hormone (FSH), which are crucial for stimulating testosterone production and maintaining healthy sperm production. Over time, this suppression can lead to testicular atrophy and a significant decrease in sperm count, a condition known as oligospermia, which can result in infertility.

Furthermore, prolonged testosterone supplementation can have a profound impact on mental health. Testosterone plays a role in mood regulation, and its imbalances are often linked to mood swings, irritability, and even depression. Users may experience heightened aggression, often referred to colloquially as 'roid rage,' a state characterized by uncontrollable anger and aggression. This altered state can strain personal relationships and lead to socially disruptive behaviors.

The cardiovascular system is another major area of concern. As discussed previously in the context of anabolic steroids, excess testosterone can lead to an increase in LDL cholesterol and a decrease in HDL cholesterol, contributing to the development of atherosclerosis. This condition narrows and hardens the arteries, increasing the risk of heart attack and stroke. Additionally, testosterone supplementation can lead to hypertension, exacerbating the risk of cardiovascular diseases.

Metabolically, prolonged use of testosterone can have significant implications. It can lead to insulin resistance, a precursor to type 2 diabetes. This resistance impairs the body's ability to regulate blood sugar levels effectively, posing long-term health risks such as kidney disease, nerve damage, and vision problems. Furthermore, testosterone can promote an increase in red blood cell production, leading to polycythemia, a condition characterized by an excessive concentration of red blood cells. While this might seem beneficial in enhancing oxygen transport, it actually increases the viscosity of the blood, making it more prone to clotting and thereby elevating the risk of thrombotic events like deep vein thrombosis or pulmonary embolism.

The musculoskeletal system is also impacted. Testosterone is known for its role in building muscle mass and strength. However, its supplementation can lead to musculoskeletal issues over time. The accelerated muscle growth can outpace the development of tendons and ligaments, leading to an increased risk of injuries such as muscle tears and tendon ruptures. Additionally, in adolescents, testosterone supplementation can prematurely close the growth plates in bones, leading to stunted growth.

Lastly, the risk of liver damage cannot be overlooked. Oral testosterone supplements, especially those that are alkylated, can be toxic to the liver. Prolonged use can lead to liver inflammation, hepatic tumors, and even liver failure. This risk is heightened when testosterone is used in combination with other substances, such as alcohol or hepatotoxic medications.

The long-term health risks associated with prolonged testosterone supplementation are multifaceted and significant. They encompass a range of physiological systems, from hormonal to cardiovascular, metabolic, musculoskeletal, and mental health. The allure of immediate benefits like enhanced muscle mass and vitality can obscure these risks, leading individuals down a path of serious and potentially irreversible health issues. It is imperative for those considering testosterone supplementation to understand these risks and for healthcare providers to diligently monitor and counsel their patients regarding the safe and appropriate use of these hormones. The pursuit of enhanced physical or sexual performance should never come at the cost of one's long-term health and well-being.

Long-term Effects on Hormonal Regulation

The disruption of the endocrine system due to long-term testosterone therapy presents a complex and multifaceted issue, deeply ingrained in the delicate balance of the body's hormonal regulation. The endocrine system, an intricate network of glands and hormones, orchestrates a multitude of bodily functions, ranging from metabolism to growth, and even emotional responses. This system, akin to a symphonic orchestra, demands precise coordination and balance for optimal functioning. Introducing external testosterone into this system can be likened to adding an uninvited musician to the orchestra, disrupting the harmony and potentially leading to a cacophony of health issues.

Long-term testosterone therapy, particularly when used without medical necessity, can significantly alter this hormonal equilibrium. The body, in its remarkable adaptive capacity, responds to the influx of external testosterone by reducing its natural production. This feedback mechanism, while efficient, can lead to a dependency on external hormones, rendering the body's own production insufficient when therapy is discontinued. The consequences of this hormonal imbalance are far-reaching and can affect various aspects of health.

One notable impact is on the reproductive system. In men, prolonged use of testosterone therapy can lead to a decrease in sperm production, testicular shrinkage, and even infertility. This occurs because the external testosterone signals the brain to reduce the production of gonadotropin-releasing hormone (GnRH), which in turn diminishes the production of the hormones necessary for sperm generation. Women, although less commonly subjected to testosterone therapy, can experience menstrual irregularities and other reproductive issues.

Another critical concern lies in the potential for exacerbating or initiating endocrine disorders. Conditions such as hypogonadism, where the body produces insufficient testosterone, can be masked by testosterone therapy, leading to delayed diagnosis and treatment. Moreover, individuals with undiagnosed or poorly managed endocrine conditions, such as thyroid disorders or adrenal gland problems, may experience worsening symptoms due to the added hormonal imbalance caused by testosterone therapy.

The psychological ramifications of this disruption should not be overlooked. Hormonal imbalances can influence mood, cognition, and overall mental health. Patients undergoing long-term testosterone therapy might experience mood swings, irritability, or even depressive symptoms as their bodies struggle to adapt to the hormonal changes. These psychological effects are not merely transient; they can have a profound and lasting impact on an individual's quality of life.

Furthermore, the endocrine system's influence on metabolic processes means that testosterone therapy can lead to unexpected metabolic changes. These can include alterations in cholesterol levels, insulin sensitivity, and body fat distribution, potentially increasing the risk of cardiovascular diseases and type 2 diabetes.

The long-term effects of testosterone therapy on the body's hormonal regulation are profound and multifaceted. They highlight the critical importance of approaching hormone therapy with caution, thorough understanding, and respect for the body's complex endocrine system. As we continue to explore the implications of hormone therapy, it is paramount that we balance the immediate benefits with a deep consideration of the potential long-term impacts on the delicate hormonal harmony that governs our health and well-being.

Age-Related Risks

The exploration of age-related risks in testosterone therapy unveils a landscape where the side effects diverge significantly between younger and older users, underscoring the complex interplay between age, hormonal balance, and health. In younger individuals, the body's natural testosterone production is typically at its peak, a period where the hormonal balance is finely tuned to support growth, muscle development, and a plethora of physiological processes. In contrast, older individuals often experience a natural decline in testosterone levels, a condition sometimes referred to as late-onset hypogonadism. This divergence in natural testosterone levels sets the stage for a varied response to testosterone therapy across different age groups.

For younger users, particularly those without a medically justifiable reason for therapy, the introduction of exogenous testosterone can disrupt the natural hormonal cycle significantly. This disruption can manifest in several ways, chief among them being the impact on fertility. Testosterone therapy in young men can lead to a decrease in sperm production, a consequence of the body's feedback mechanism that reduces the production of gonadotropins, hormones essential for sperm generation. Additionally, young users may experience premature closing of the growth plates in bones, potentially stunting growth if therapy is initiated before the completion of puberty.

Psychological effects also tend to be more pronounced in younger individuals. Testosterone is not merely a physical hormone; it plays a crucial role in mental and emotional health. Young adults, often still in the process of emotional and psychological development, might find themselves grappling with exacerbated aggression, mood swings, or other behavioral changes. These effects, while concerning at any age, can be particularly disruptive during the formative years of young adulthood.

In older users, the risks of testosterone therapy take on a different hue. The most prominent concern lies in the cardiovascular realm. Older adults, particularly those with pre-existing cardiovascular conditions, may face an increased risk of heart attacks, strokes, and other cardiac events as a result of testosterone therapy. This risk is attributed to various factors, including the potential for testosterone to increase blood viscosity and alter cholesterol levels.

Another significant risk for older individuals is the impact on prostate health. Testosterone can stimulate the growth of the prostate gland, and in individuals with undiagnosed prostate cancer, therapy could accelerate the progression of the disease. Moreover, even in the absence of cancer, an enlarged prostate can lead to urinary difficulties and other discomforts.

Bone density changes also present a unique risk in the older population. While testosterone can help maintain bone density, the imbalance caused by therapy might lead to an increased risk of osteoporosis and fractures, especially if therapy is abruptly discontinued.

The age-related risks associated with testosterone therapy underscore the need for a personalized and cautious approach. Younger users face risks primarily related to fertility, growth, and psychological effects, while older users are more susceptible to cardiovascular issues, prostate health concerns, and bone density changes. These differences highlight the importance of considering age as a crucial factor in the decision-making process surrounding testosterone therapy, ensuring that the benefits and risks are carefully weighed to safeguard the health and well-being of each individual.

Gender-Specific Concerns

The gender-specific concerns associated with testosterone therapy reveal a nuanced landscape of risks, unique to men and women, that underscore the complex nature of hormonal treatments. In men, testosterone therapy is more commonly prescribed, often aimed at addressing issues like hypogonadism, where the body's natural testosterone production is insufficient. For women, testosterone therapy is less common and typically focused on specific medical conditions or as part of a broader hormone replacement therapy.

In men, one of the primary concerns with testosterone therapy is its impact on fertility. Testosterone plays a crucial role in spermatogenesis, the process of sperm production. Paradoxically, while it is essential for sperm production, excessive levels of externally administered testosterone can lead to a significant reduction in sperm count. This occurs because the introduction of external testosterone disrupts the body's natural feedback mechanism, reducing the production of gonadotropin-releasing hormone (GnRH) and consequently lowering the levels of follicle-stimulating hormone (FSH) and luteinizing hormone (LH), both of which are critical for sperm production. This effect can be temporary or, in some cases, lead to long-term or permanent fertility issues.

Another major concern for men is the potential exacerbation of prostate health issues. Testosterone can stimulate the growth of the prostate gland. In cases of undiagnosed prostate cancer, testosterone therapy could accelerate the cancer's progression. Additionally, an enlarged prostate, even in the absence of malignancy, can lead to urinary difficulties and discomfort.

For women, testosterone therapy is typically less common and is often part of a broader approach to treating certain health conditions, such as breast cancer or as a component of menopausal hormone therapy. The risks in women are distinct and less well-understood, owing to the lower frequency of use and a historical focus on men in testosterone research. However, it's known that excessive testosterone in women can lead to a range of side effects, including virilization, which encompasses symptoms such as deepening of the voice, increased body hair, and changes in menstrual cycles. These effects can be distressing and, in some cases, irreversible, making the decision to commence testosterone therapy in women a complex and carefully considered one.

In both men and women, there are also risks related to cardiovascular health. Testosterone therapy can influence cholesterol levels, blood viscosity, and overall cardiovascular function. These effects can increase the risk of heart attacks and strokes, particularly in individuals with pre-existing cardiovascular conditions.

Moreover, the psychological and emotional impacts of testosterone therapy can be significant for both genders. Alterations in mood, increases in aggression, and other psychological effects have been observed. These changes can be particularly pronounced in individuals with pre-existing mental health conditions.

The gender-specific concerns related to testosterone therapy are multifaceted and require a tailored approach. In men, the primary risks revolve around fertility, prostate health, and cardiovascular issues. For women, concerns include virilization, menstrual irregularities, and potentially under-researched cardiovascular risks. These distinctions highlight the need for gender-specific research, careful patient evaluation, and personalized treatment plans to mitigate risks and ensure the safe and effective use of testosterone therapy.

Pre-existing Conditions

When delving into the realm of testosterone therapy and pre-existing conditions, we uncover a complex interplay where this treatment can potentially exacerbate certain health issues, adding layers of risk and consideration to an already intricate medical decision. Testosterone, a hormone pivotal in numerous physiological processes, does not operate in isolation within the body. Its effects are widespread and can significantly influence pre-existing medical conditions, sometimes aggravating them or triggering new complications.

One of the most critical concerns surrounds cardiovascular health. Testosterone therapy has been linked to an increased risk of cardiovascular events, such as heart attacks and strokes. This risk is particularly heightened in individuals with a history of heart disease or risk factors such as hypertension, high cholesterol, or atherosclerosis. The mechanism behind this increased risk is multifaceted, involving changes in cholesterol levels, blood viscosity, and possibly direct effects on the heart muscle and blood vessels. For patients with pre-existing cardiovascular conditions, testosterone therapy can thus act as a catalyst, potentially accelerating the progression of their heart disease.

Another significant area of concern is prostate health in men. Testosterone can stimulate the growth of the prostate gland, and in cases of undiagnosed prostate cancer, it may hasten the cancer's development. Even benign enlargement of the prostate, a common condition in older men, can be exacerbated by testosterone therapy, leading to urinary difficulties and discomfort. This makes a thorough evaluation of prostate health a vital component of the decision-making process when considering testosterone therapy.

For individuals with liver disease, testosterone therapy poses additional risks. Testosterone and its metabolites can be taxing on the liver, potentially exacerbating existing liver conditions such as cirrhosis or fatty liver disease. This is especially concerning when considering oral testosterone preparations, which have been shown to have a more pronounced impact on liver function.

Endocrine disorders also merit special attention in the context of testosterone therapy. Conditions like hypogonadism, thyroid disorders, and adrenal insufficiency are all intricately linked to the body's hormonal milieu. Introducing external testosterone can upset this balance, potentially masking symptoms of these conditions or complicating their management. Particularly in cases of hypogonadism, distinguishing between primary (testicular) and secondary (pituitary or hypothalamic) causes is crucial, as testosterone therapy may be inappropriate and even harmful in certain types of secondary hypogonadism.

Mental health conditions are another domain where testosterone therapy can have profound implications. While testosterone can influence mood and cognitive function, in individuals with pre-existing mental health disorders, such as depression, anxiety, or bipolar disorder, it can exacerbate symptoms or lead to new mental health challenges. The hormonal fluctuations induced by therapy can significantly impact emotional and psychological well-being, necessitating careful monitoring and management.

The consideration of pre-existing conditions is paramount in the context of testosterone therapy. Cardiovascular disease, prostate health, liver function, endocrine disorders, and mental health are all intricately affected by testosterone levels. This necessitates a holistic and comprehensive approach to patient evaluation and monitoring, ensuring that the potential benefits of therapy are carefully weighed against the risks posed to existing health issues. It underscores the importance of personalized medicine, where treatment decisions are made not just on the basis of a single hormone level, but in the context of the patient's entire health profile.

Mental Health Risks

The intersection of testosterone therapy and mental health presents a nuanced and complex picture, where the hormonal intervention can influence, and sometimes exacerbate, mental health conditions such as depression, anxiety, and other disorders. The intricate relationship between hormones and mental health is well-established, yet the specific impacts of testosterone therapy on psychological well-being remain a topic of significant clinical interest and debate. Testosterone, often dubbed the "male" hormone, is not merely a physical entity; it plays a substantial role in emotional regulation and cognitive function, thus making its supplementation a matter of delicate consideration, particularly for individuals with pre-existing mental health concerns.

Depression, a prevalent mental health disorder characterized by persistent sadness, loss of interest, and a myriad of physical and emotional symptoms, can have a complex relationship with testosterone levels. Some studies suggest that low testosterone levels are associated with increased symptoms of depression in men, leading to the hypothesis that testosterone therapy could potentially alleviate these symptoms. However, the reality is far more intricate. While some individuals may experience an improvement in mood and emotional well-being with testosterone therapy, others might find their symptoms of depression exacerbated. The reasons for these divergent outcomes are not entirely clear but are thought to involve individual differences in brain chemistry, hormone receptors, and the underlying causes of depression.

Anxiety disorders, marked by excessive worry, fear, and a range of physical symptoms such as heart palpitations and restlessness, also enter into a complex dance with testosterone therapy. Testosterone can influence the body's stress response system, potentially affecting the prevalence and severity of anxiety symptoms. For some individuals, testosterone supplementation can lead to heightened anxiety, possibly due to the hormone's effects on neurochemistry and the stress response system. Conversely, others may find a reduction in anxiety symptoms, perhaps due to the improved energy levels and sense of well-being that can accompany balanced testosterone levels.

Beyond depression and anxiety, testosterone therapy can impact a range of other mental health disorders. For instance, it has been observed to influence mood regulation, sometimes leading to increased irritability, aggression, or mood swings. This is particularly relevant in individuals with bipolar disorder or other mood disorders, where the introduction of testosterone can destabilize mood and exacerbate the cyclic nature of these conditions.

It is also critical to consider the psychological aspect of dependence and the mental health implications of long-term hormone supplementation. Individuals undergoing testosterone therapy, particularly those who start it without clear medical indications, can develop a psychological dependence on the hormone, believing it to be essential for their well-being and confidence. This dependence can lead to challenges in discontinuing therapy, including withdrawal symptoms that mimic or exacerbate mental health disorders.

The potential mental health risks associated with testosterone therapy are significant and multifaceted. They highlight the necessity for a careful and comprehensive approach to mental health evaluation both before and during testosterone therapy. Clinicians must be vigilant in monitoring for changes in mood, anxiety levels, and other psychiatric symptoms, tailoring therapy to the individual's needs and adjusting or discontinuing treatment as necessary. For patients, it is crucial to approach testosterone therapy with an understanding of these potential risks and to maintain open and ongoing communication with healthcare providers about any changes in mental health. This conscientious approach ensures that the benefits of testosterone therapy are balanced against the potential for exacerbating existing mental health conditions or triggering new psychiatric symptoms.

Behavioral Changes

The realm of testosterone therapy and its impact on behavior opens a window into a world where subtle hormonal shifts can lead to significant changes in aggression, risk-taking behavior, and interpersonal relationships. Testosterone, a hormone deeply intertwined with physical and psychological processes, does not limit its influence to mere physiological functions. Its role in shaping behavior has been a subject of interest and research for decades, revealing a complex and sometimes controversial connection between hormone levels and behavioral patterns. In the context of testosterone therapy, particularly when administered without strict medical necessity, this connection becomes even more pronounced and consequential.

Aggression, often linked to testosterone in both scientific and popular discourse, is a multifaceted behavioral change that can be influenced by testosterone therapy. The hormone has been associated with increased assertiveness and, in some cases, aggressive behavior. This link, however, is not straightforward. While some individuals may experience heightened aggression or irritability as a result of testosterone supplementation, others may not notice significant changes in their behavior. The variability in response is thought to be due to individual differences in biology, psychology, and social conditioning. In some cases, the increase in aggressive behavior can be subtle, manifesting as a lowered threshold for frustration or a heightened response to perceived challenges. In others, it can be more pronounced, leading to overtly aggressive actions or conflicts.

Risk-taking behavior is another area where testosterone therapy can have a notable impact. Testosterone has been associated with increased risk-taking tendencies, a trait that can manifest in various aspects of life, from financial decisions to physical activities. The mechanism behind this effect is thought to involve testosterone's influence on the brain's reward system, potentially leading to a heightened sense of confidence and a diminished perception of risk. This altered risk assessment can have profound implications, not just for the individual undergoing therapy, but also for their professional and personal lives.

The impact of testosterone therapy on relationships is perhaps one of the most significant yet underappreciated aspects of behavioral change. Relationships, whether romantic, familial, or social, are built on a foundation of emotional connection, communication, and mutual understanding. Changes in behavior, such as increased aggression or risk-taking, can strain these connections, leading to conflicts, misunderstandings, and a disruption in the dynamic of relationships. For romantic partners, these changes can be particularly challenging, as they may affect intimacy, communication, and the overall emotional climate of the relationship. Similarly, altered behavior can impact parenting styles, friendships, and professional relationships, altering the way an individual interacts with the world around them.

The behavioral changes associated with testosterone therapy, including increased aggression, heightened risk-taking behavior, and the impact on relationships, are significant and warrant careful consideration. These changes highlight the need for a holistic approach to testosterone therapy, one that not only addresses the physiological aspects but also takes into account the psychological and social dimensions. Patients and healthcare providers must be vigilant in monitoring these behavioral changes, engaging in open communication about any shifts in behavior, and adjusting therapy as needed. This approach ensures that the potential benefits of testosterone therapy are not overshadowed by unintended and potentially disruptive changes in behavior.

Dependency and Withdrawal

The issues of dependency and withdrawal in the context of long-term testosterone therapy present a critical aspect of the treatment that requires careful consideration. Testosterone therapy, particularly when used over extended periods, can lead to a complex relationship between the body and the hormone, characterized by dependency and challenging withdrawal symptoms upon cessation. This dynamic underscores the importance of understanding and managing the long-term implications of testosterone supplementation, beyond its immediate effects.

Dependency on testosterone therapy can manifest in both physiological and psychological forms. Physiologically, the body may become accustomed to the external supply of testosterone, leading to a reduction in its natural production. The endocrine system, particularly the hypothalamic-pituitary-gonadal axis, which regulates natural testosterone production, can become suppressed. This suppression means that when testosterone therapy is discontinued, the body may not immediately resume its normal hormone production, leading to a period of hormonal imbalance. Symptoms of low testosterone, such as fatigue, reduced libido, and decreased muscle mass, can re-emerge, often more acutely than before the therapy was initiated.

Psychological dependency is also a significant concern. Individuals undergoing testosterone therapy may experience an enhanced sense of well-being, increased energy, and improved physical performance while on the therapy. These positive effects can lead to a psychological reliance on the hormone, where the individual feels dependent on testosterone for maintaining their quality of life. This reliance can make the prospect of discontinuing therapy daunting, leading to hesitation or refusal to stop treatment even when medically advisable.

Withdrawal symptoms are a key issue when ceasing testosterone therapy, especially after long-term use. These symptoms can be both physical and psychological. Physically, individuals may experience fatigue, weakness, weight gain, and a return of symptoms that were initially treated by the therapy, such as erectile dysfunction or decreased bone density. Psychologically, withdrawal can lead to mood swings, irritability, depression, and a sense of decreased mental clarity. The severity and duration of these symptoms can vary widely among individuals, influenced by factors such as the duration of therapy, the dosage used, and individual physiological differences.

Managing these issues of dependency and withdrawal requires a thoughtful and strategic approach. Gradual tapering of the hormone, rather than abrupt cessation, can help mitigate withdrawal symptoms and allow the body time to resume natural testosterone production. Monitoring and support during the withdrawal phase are crucial, with attention given to both physical and mental health. In some cases, supplemental therapies or medications may be needed to manage specific symptoms of withdrawal.

The issues of dependency and withdrawal in long-term testosterone therapy are significant concerns that necessitate careful planning and management. Recognizing the potential for physiological and psychological dependency is essential, as is preparing for and managing the withdrawal process. A collaborative approach involving the patient and healthcare provider, with a focus on gradual adjustment and comprehensive support, can help ensure a safe and effective transition off testosterone therapy. This approach underscores the importance of viewing testosterone therapy as a component of a broader health management strategy, rather than a standalone treatment, ensuring that the long-term health and well-being of the patient remain the central focus.

Social Pressure and Body Image

The influence of social pressure and body image on the decision to use testosterone therapy opens a window into the broader cultural and societal factors that shape our health choices. In a world where physical appearance and athletic performance are often highly valued, the allure of testosterone therapy as a means to enhance muscle mass, increase energy, and improve overall physical prowess can be compelling. This societal backdrop, marked by an emphasis on youthfulness, strength, and vitality, plays a significant role in shaping perceptions and decisions regarding hormone therapy, often blurring the line between medical necessity and the pursuit of an idealized body image.

The impact of social pressure on the decision to use testosterone therapy is particularly evident in the realm of body image. The contemporary ideal of masculinity, often portrayed in media and popular culture, emphasizes muscularity, leanness, and physical strength. For many men, this ideal can feel unattainable or may push them to pursue physical enhancements through artificial means, including testosterone therapy. The hormone's association with increased muscle mass, reduced body fat, and improved energy levels makes it an attractive option for those seeking to conform to these societal standards. However, this pursuit is not without risks, as the use of testosterone therapy for non-medical purposes can lead to significant health complications.

In addition to the influence on men, societal norms and body image pressures can also affect women's decisions regarding testosterone therapy. While less commonly discussed, the use of testosterone in women, particularly in the context of athletic performance or bodybuilding, reflects a similar response to societal pressures around physical appearance and performance. Women may turn to testosterone for its muscle-building and fat-reducing effects, driven by a culture that increasingly values athleticism and strength in female bodies.

The role of social media and advertising in perpetuating these body image ideals cannot be overlooked. Marketing campaigns often present testosterone therapy as a panacea for aging-related issues, weight gain, and decreased libido, playing into societal fears of aging and loss of vitality. This marketing is powerful and pervasive, shaping public perceptions about the necessity and benefits of hormone therapy, often without adequately addressing the potential risks and long-term health implications.

Addressing the role of social pressure and body image in decisions about testosterone therapy requires a multi-faceted approach. Healthcare providers play a crucial role in educating patients about the appropriate use of testosterone therapy, distinguishing between medical needs and the desire to achieve a certain physical aesthetic. It's important for individuals considering therapy to engage in a thorough evaluation of their motivations, informed by an understanding of the risks and benefits.

The impact of social pressure and body image on the decision to use testosterone therapy is a significant aspect of the broader conversation about hormone use. The societal idealization of certain body types and physical attributes can drive individuals to pursue testosterone therapy for non-medical reasons, a choice that carries potential health risks. Recognizing and addressing these societal influences is essential in ensuring that decisions about testosterone therapy are made based on medical need and a comprehensive understanding of the risks and benefits, rather than solely on cultural ideals and external pressures.

Ethical Considerations

The ethical considerations surrounding the prescription and management of testosterone therapy by healthcare providers delve into a realm where medical responsibility intersects with patient autonomy and well-being. In an era where hormone treatments are increasingly sought after for both medical and non-medical reasons, the role of healthcare providers becomes pivotal in navigating the complex ethical landscape of testosterone therapy. This responsibility encompasses not only the appropriate prescription and management of the therapy but also involves educating patients, managing expectations, and safeguarding against potential misuse.

One of the primary ethical responsibilities of healthcare providers is to ensure that testosterone therapy is prescribed appropriately and judiciously. This means conducting a thorough evaluation to ascertain whether a patient truly has a medical condition that warrants testosterone supplementation, such as hypogonadism, rather than prescribing it for non-medical reasons like anti-aging or purely for enhancing physical appearance or athletic performance. Accurate diagnosis requires careful consideration of symptoms, along with appropriate testing to confirm low testosterone levels. This approach respects the principle of "do no harm," ensuring that the potential benefits of therapy outweigh the risks for each individual patient.

Another key ethical consideration is informed consent. Patients must be fully informed about the potential risks and benefits of testosterone therapy, including the possibility of side effects, long-term health implications, and the potential need for lifelong treatment. This information should be communicated clearly and without bias, allowing patients to make an informed decision about their treatment. Healthcare providers must also be vigilant in identifying and addressing any misconceptions or unrealistic expectations that patients may have about the therapy, often influenced by media portrayals and societal pressures.

The management of testosterone therapy also presents ethical challenges. Providers must monitor patients closely, adjusting treatment as necessary to minimize risks and optimize outcomes. This includes regular follow-ups to assess hormone levels, evaluate side effects, and ensure that the therapy is achieving its intended goals. For patients who wish to discontinue therapy, providers should offer guidance and support, helping them to manage withdrawal symptoms and adjust to changes in their hormone levels.

There is also an ethical imperative to consider broader societal implications, such as the impact on health disparities and access to care. Testosterone therapy, like many specialized treatments, can be expensive and not always covered by insurance, potentially creating barriers to access for some populations. Healthcare providers must be cognizant of these disparities and strive to provide equitable care, ensuring that decisions about therapy are not unduly influenced by a patient's socio-economic status.

The ethical considerations in prescribing and managing testosterone therapy place significant responsibility on healthcare providers. They must ensure appropriate use, provide thorough patient education, manage therapy effectively, and consider broader societal implications. Upholding these ethical standards is crucial in ensuring that testosterone therapy is used safely and effectively, prioritizing the health and well-being of patients while navigating the complex and evolving landscape of hormone treatments.

Regulatory Oversight

Current policies, implemented by regulatory bodies such as the Food and Drug Administration (FDA) and similar organizations globally, are designed to oversee the prescription, distribution, and monitoring of testosterone products. These policies play a pivotal role in safeguarding patients, although their effectiveness can vary and is subject to ongoing evaluation and necessary adaptation in response to emerging data and trends.

One of the primary functions of regulatory oversight is to control the approval and distribution of testosterone products. This involves a rigorous process of evaluating the safety and efficacy of testosterone formulations before they can be made available to the public. Manufacturers are required to conduct clinical trials and submit detailed data demonstrating that their products are both safe and effective for their intended use. This process is designed to prevent the introduction of unsafe or ineffective treatments into the market, although it is not infallible and is often a subject of debate and scrutiny.

Another key aspect of regulatory oversight is the creation and enforcement of guidelines for prescribing testosterone therapy. These guidelines are based on current medical research and expert consensus, aiming to standardize treatment practices and reduce the risk of inappropriate prescribing. They typically include criteria for diagnosing conditions like hypogonadism, recommendations for dosing and monitoring, and guidance on managing side effects. While these guidelines are valuable in promoting best practices, their effectiveness depends heavily on the extent to which healthcare providers adhere to them.

Regulatory bodies also play a role in monitoring the long-term safety of testosterone products. This involves post-marketing surveillance to track adverse events and other safety concerns that may emerge once a product is used by the general population. Such surveillance is critical in identifying rare or delayed side effects that may not have been apparent in clinical trials. However, this system relies on the reporting of adverse events, which can be inconsistent, leading to potential underestimation of risks.

One of the challenges in regulatory oversight of testosterone therapy is addressing the issue of off-label use. While healthcare providers are allowed to prescribe medications for off-label purposes (uses not specifically approved by regulatory bodies), this practice can lead to scenarios where patients receive testosterone therapy without a clear medical indication. Regulating and monitoring off-label use is complex and requires a balance between allowing physician discretion and ensuring patient safety.

In addition to these measures, regulatory bodies often engage in public education efforts, providing information about the appropriate use of testosterone therapy and its potential risks. This is particularly important given the influence of direct-to-consumer advertising and other marketing strategies that can shape public perceptions and demand for testosterone products.

The regulatory oversight of testosterone therapy involves multiple strategies aimed at ensuring the safety and efficacy of treatments, standardizing prescribing practices, monitoring long-term safety, and educating the public. While current policies play a crucial role in safeguarding patients, their effectiveness is contingent upon continuous evaluation, adaptation to new evidence, and effective enforcement. This dynamic and multifaceted approach is essential in addressing the challenges posed by testosterone therapy and ensuring that its benefits are delivered within a framework of patient safety and well-being.

The Regulatory Landscape

The regulatory landscape governing testosterone prescriptions is an intricate and evolving framework designed to ensure the safe and effective use of this hormone therapy. This landscape is shaped by a variety of regulatory bodies, guidelines, and legal requirements, each playing a crucial role in how testosterone is prescribed and managed in the healthcare setting. The overarching goal of these regulations is to safeguard patient health, prevent misuse, and ensure that testosterone therapy is used appropriately, based on sound medical evidence.

At the forefront of this regulatory framework in many countries, including the United States, is the Food and Drug Administration (FDA) or equivalent national regulatory agencies. These bodies are responsible for the approval of testosterone products, a process that involves a rigorous review of clinical trial data to assess the safety and efficacy of the hormone for specific conditions. This approval process is critical in determining which testosterone formulations are available on the market and for what indications they can be used.

In addition to product approval, these agencies also establish guidelines for the prescribing of testosterone. These guidelines are based on the latest clinical research and expert consensus, and they provide healthcare providers with criteria for diagnosing conditions like hypogonadism, which is a key indication for testosterone therapy. The guidelines also cover recommended dosages, administration methods, and monitoring protocols to ensure that patients receive the most appropriate and effective treatment. Adherence to these guidelines is crucial for healthcare providers to ensure they are delivering care that aligns with the current standards of medical practice.

The regulatory landscape also includes mechanisms for monitoring the safety of testosterone products once they are on the market. This post-market surveillance is vital for identifying any adverse effects or safety concerns that might arise when the products are used by a broader patient population outside of clinical trials. This surveillance often involves the reporting of adverse events by healthcare providers and patients, which regulatory agencies review to determine if additional warnings, usage restrictions, or even product withdrawals are necessary.

Control of advertising and marketing of testosterone products is another important aspect of the regulatory framework. In many countries, there are strict rules governing how pharmaceutical companies can promote their products, particularly in direct-to-consumer advertising. These regulations are intended to ensure that promotional materials are not misleading, overstate the benefits, or understate the risks of testosterone therapy. Effective regulation of marketing is crucial to prevent the creation of unrealistic expectations or inappropriate demand among potential patients.

In some regions, there are also legal requirements and restrictions on testosterone due to its potential for abuse, given its performance-enhancing effects. Testosterone is classified as a controlled substance in many countries, meaning its prescription and distribution are subject to additional oversight and restrictions. This classification aims to prevent misuse and diversion of the hormone for non-medical purposes, such as athletic performance enhancement or bodybuilding.

The regulatory landscape governing testosterone prescriptions is, therefore, a complex and multi-layered system that involves product approval, prescribing guidelines, post-marketing surveillance, marketing control, and legal classification. This system is continually evolving in response to new scientific evidence, changes in medical practice, and emerging safety information, reflecting the dynamic nature of healthcare regulation. It underscores the importance of a balanced approach that ensures access to testosterone therapy for those who need it, while minimizing the risks of misuse, adverse effects, and inappropriate prescribing.

Emerging Research

The landscape of hormone therapy, particularly regarding testosterone, is an area of dynamic and ongoing research, with emerging studies continually shaping our understanding and approach to treatment. The future directions in hormone therapy research are driven by a quest to enhance efficacy, reduce risks, and broaden the understanding of hormonal impacts on various aspects of health. This evolving field holds promise for more personalized, safe, and effective hormonal treatments, reflecting the advancements in medical science and technology.

One key area of emerging research is the development of new testosterone delivery systems. Current methods, such as injections, patches, gels, and pills, each have their limitations and side effects. Researchers are exploring novel delivery mechanisms, like long-acting injectables or implantable devices, that could provide more stable hormone levels and reduce the frequency of administration. There is also interest in developing formulations that minimize fluctuations in testosterone levels, thereby reducing side effects and improving patient outcomes.

Another significant area of research is the investigation into the long-term effects of testosterone therapy. While current knowledge provides insight into the short-term benefits and risks of testosterone treatment, there is a need for more comprehensive data on its long-term impact, particularly regarding cardiovascular health, prostate cancer risk, and mental health. Longitudinal studies and large-scale clinical trials are required to better understand these long-term outcomes and to refine treatment guidelines accordingly.

Personalized hormone therapy is also a burgeoning field of interest. This approach involves tailoring hormone treatments based on individual patient factors, such as genetic makeup, existing health conditions, and specific symptoms. Advances in genomics and precision medicine could enable healthcare providers to predict how individual patients might respond to testosterone therapy, allowing for more personalized and effective treatment plans.

Furthermore, there is a growing interest in exploring the broader applications of testosterone therapy beyond traditional uses. This includes research into the use of testosterone for conditions like muscle wasting diseases, certain forms of breast cancer, or major depressive disorder. Investigating the potential benefits of testosterone in these areas could lead to new therapeutic applications and a better understanding of the hormone's multifaceted roles in the body.

The impact of testosterone therapy on different populations is also a critical area of research. Much of the existing data is based on studies in middle-aged and older men. There is a need for more research on the effects of testosterone therapy in women, younger men, and individuals of different ethnic backgrounds to ensure that treatment guidelines are applicable and safe for a diverse patient population.

Finally, the ethical and societal implications of hormone therapy, including testosterone treatment, continue to be an important area of study. This includes examining the impact of societal attitudes on treatment decisions, the ethical considerations in prescribing hormone therapy, and the regulatory challenges associated with new and existing treatments.

Emerging research and future directions in hormone therapy are focused on developing new delivery methods, understanding long-term effects, personalizing treatment approaches, exploring broader therapeutic applications, studying impacts on diverse populations, and addressing ethical and societal issues. These research endeavors hold the potential to significantly advance the field of hormone therapy, leading to improved patient outcomes and a deeper understanding of hormonal health.

Testosterone Therapy Safety

Navigating testosterone therapy safely involves a set of comprehensive guidelines and best practices for both patients and healthcare providers. These guidelines are crucial in ensuring that the use of testosterone therapy is not only effective but also minimizes risks and potential side effects. In the evolving field of hormone therapy, adherence to these practices is key to achieving the best possible outcomes for patients.

For healthcare providers, the first step in ensuring safe use of testosterone therapy is a thorough and accurate diagnosis. This involves confirming low testosterone levels through reliable laboratory tests and assessing whether the patient's symptoms align with a medical need for testosterone supplementation. It's essential to rule out other potential causes of the patient's symptoms and to consider their overall health and medical history, including any pre-existing conditions that might be contraindicated with testosterone therapy.

Once therapy is deemed necessary, healthcare providers should prescribe the lowest effective dose of testosterone to achieve the desired therapeutic goals. This approach minimizes the risk of side effects and complications. It's also important to choose the appropriate delivery method (injections, patches, gels, or other formulations) based on the patient's lifestyle, preference, and medical considerations.

Regular monitoring is a critical aspect of safe testosterone therapy. Healthcare providers should schedule follow-up appointments to monitor the patient's hormone levels, adjust dosages as necessary, and evaluate for side effects. These appointments are also opportunities to assess the therapy's effectiveness and make any necessary adjustments to the treatment plan.

Patient education is another cornerstone of safe testosterone therapy. Patients should be fully informed about the potential risks and benefits of the therapy, how to properly administer the treatment, and what side effects to look out for. They should also be educated on the importance of adhering to the prescribed treatment regimen and the potential consequences of misuse or overuse.

For patients, adhering to the prescribed therapy regimen is essential for safe and effective treatment. This includes taking the medication exactly as prescribed, attending all follow-up appointments, and being vigilant about monitoring for side effects. Patients should promptly report any side effects or concerns to their healthcare provider.

Lifestyle factors also play a significant role in the safe use of testosterone therapy. Patients should maintain a healthy lifestyle, including a balanced diet, regular exercise, and avoiding excessive alcohol and tobacco use, as these can affect hormone levels and the overall effectiveness of the therapy.

In the case of patients looking to discontinue testosterone therapy, it's important to do so under the guidance of a healthcare provider. Abrupt cessation can lead to withdrawal symptoms and a rebound effect. A gradual tapering off, as advised by the healthcare provider, is usually the safest approach.

Finally, patients should be aware of the legal and ethical considerations surrounding testosterone therapy, particularly the risks associated with obtaining and using testosterone without a prescription or for non-medical reasons.

The safe use of testosterone therapy hinges on accurate diagnosis, appropriate prescription, regular monitoring, patient education, adherence to treatment, a healthy lifestyle, and careful discontinuation under medical supervision. Both patients and healthcare providers have crucial roles to play in ensuring that testosterone therapy is used safely and effectively, with the well-being of the patient as the primary concern.

Monitoring and Managing Side Effects

Monitoring and managing side effects in testosterone therapy is a critical aspect of patient care, essential for mitigating risks and ensuring the safety and effectiveness of the treatment. Testosterone, like all hormones, has a profound impact on the body, and its supplementation can lead to a range of side effects. The key to managing these side effects lies in vigilant monitoring, early detection, and strategic interventions by both healthcare providers and patients.

For healthcare providers, the process of monitoring begins even before the initiation of therapy. A comprehensive baseline assessment, including a detailed medical history and a full spectrum of blood tests, sets the stage for understanding the patient's unique risk profile. Once therapy commences, regular follow-up appointments are crucial. These appointments should include assessments of testosterone levels and other relevant parameters such as hematocrit, cholesterol levels, liver function tests, and prostate-specific antigen (PSA) levels, depending on the patient's individual risk factors.

In addition to laboratory monitoring, healthcare providers should conduct thorough clinical evaluations at each visit. This involves discussing any physical or psychological symptoms the patient may be experiencing. Common side effects of testosterone therapy include acne, sleep apnea, polycythemia (an increase in red blood cell count), and changes in cholesterol levels. More serious side effects, though less common, can include cardiovascular events and exacerbation of prostate cancer. Early detection of these side effects is critical for timely intervention.

Patient education plays a pivotal role in managing side effects. Patients should be informed about the potential side effects of testosterone therapy and instructed on how to recognize them. Empowering patients with this knowledge enables them to be active participants in their care and increases the likelihood of early detection of side effects.

Lifestyle modifications can also be a valuable strategy in managing side effects. For example, maintaining a healthy weight, engaging in regular exercise, and following a heart-healthy diet can help mitigate cardiovascular risks. Patients should also be advised on ways to manage minor side effects at home, such as using skincare products for acne or adjusting sleep positions to alleviate mild sleep apnea.

For some side effects, medication adjustments may be necessary. This could involve altering the dose of testosterone, changing the delivery method, or introducing additional medications to counteract specific side effects. For instance, in the case of polycythemia, a reduction in the testosterone dose or therapeutic phlebotomy (blood withdrawal) might be required.

In situations where side effects are severe or pose significant health risks, discontinuation of testosterone therapy may be the safest course of action. This decision should be made collaboratively between the patient and the healthcare provider, considering the benefits of the therapy against its risks.

It's important to recognize that each patient's experience with testosterone therapy is unique. What constitutes a side effect for one individual may not be the same for another. Personalized care and an individualized approach to monitoring and managing side effects are essential.

When to Say No

Understanding when to say no to testosterone therapy is a critical decision-making aspect for both patients and healthcare providers. Testosterone therapy, while beneficial for certain medical conditions, is not suitable for everyone and can pose significant risks under certain circumstances. Recognizing the situations where the risks of testosterone therapy outweigh the potential benefits is key to making informed and safe healthcare decisions.

The first scenario where testosterone therapy might not be the right choice is when the symptoms of low testosterone are absent or minimal. Symptoms like reduced libido, fatigue, and loss of muscle strength are often attributed to low testosterone levels, but they can also be caused by a range of other factors, including stress, poor diet, lack of exercise, and other health conditions. If these symptoms are not clearly linked to clinically low testosterone levels, as determined by blood tests, then testosterone therapy may not be appropriate.

Another critical consideration is the presence of certain medical conditions. Men with a history of prostate or breast cancer should generally avoid testosterone therapy, as it can stimulate the growth of these cancers. Similarly, individuals with severe untreated sleep apnea, severe heart conditions, or uncontrolled heart failure should be cautious, as testosterone therapy can exacerbate these conditions. For patients with a history of blood clots or polycythemia (a condition characterized by an elevated red blood cell count), testosterone therapy poses additional risks and is often advised against.

Age is also a factor in deciding against testosterone therapy. In older men, particularly those with age-related decline in testosterone levels, the risks of therapy, such as cardiovascular events or exacerbation of prostate health issues, can be more pronounced. The decision to use testosterone therapy in older adults should be approached with caution, weighing the potential benefits against the increased risks.

For individuals seeking testosterone therapy for non-medical reasons, such as to enhance athletic performance, increase muscle mass, or combat natural aging processes, the decision should be a resounding no. The use of testosterone for such purposes is not only medically inappropriate but also poses significant health risks and ethical concerns.

Mental health considerations also play a role in deciding against testosterone therapy. In individuals with a history of mental health disorders, such as severe depression, bipolar disorder, or psychosis, testosterone therapy can sometimes exacerbate symptoms. A thorough mental health evaluation and discussion of the potential psychological impacts of testosterone therapy are essential in these cases.

Patient preference and lifestyle factors should not be overlooked. Some individuals may prefer to explore alternative treatments, such as lifestyle changes, dietary adjustments, or other medical therapies. The decision to decline testosterone therapy should be respected and supported, with an emphasis on exploring other avenues to address the patient's health concerns.

Natural Testosterone Management

Natural testosterone management encompasses a holistic approach that involves lifestyle modifications, dietary changes, and non-hormonal medical interventions. This approach is particularly relevant for individuals looking to naturally boost their testosterone levels without resorting to hormone therapy, or for those for whom testosterone therapy is not suitable. By focusing on natural methods, one can often improve overall health and well-being while potentially enhancing their body's natural testosterone production.

Lifestyle changes are a cornerstone of natural testosterone management. Regular physical activity, especially strength training and high-intensity interval training (HIIT), has been shown to boost testosterone levels. Exercise not only helps in maintaining a healthy weight but also aids in muscle building, both of which are associated with higher testosterone levels. Additionally, getting adequate sleep is crucial, as poor sleep patterns can significantly lower testosterone levels. Aim for 7-9 hours of quality sleep per night, as this is when the body produces the most testosterone.

Diet also plays a critical role in managing testosterone levels. Including certain foods in the diet can support the body's natural testosterone production. Foods rich in vitamin D, zinc, and omega-3 fatty acids have been linked to higher testosterone levels. Examples include fatty fish like salmon and mackerel, leafy green vegetables, nuts and seeds, and eggs. On the other hand, a diet high in processed foods, excessive sugar, and trans fats can lead to lower testosterone levels and should be avoided.

Reducing stress is another key element in natural testosterone management. Chronic stress leads to prolonged elevations in cortisol, a hormone that can negatively affect testosterone levels. Engaging in stress-reduction techniques such as meditation, yoga, deep breathing exercises, or even pursuing hobbies can help in managing stress effectively.

Non-hormonal medical interventions can also play a role. For instance, certain medications and supplements, though not directly testosterone-based, can help in improving testosterone levels or counteracting the symptoms of low testosterone. Supplements like vitamin D, zinc, and magnesium may be beneficial, but it's important to consult with a healthcare provider before starting any supplementation, as overuse or incorrect supplementation can have adverse effects.

In addition to these lifestyle and dietary interventions, regular medical check-ups are important. These can help identify and manage any underlying health issues that might be contributing to low testosterone levels, such as obesity, diabetes, or hormonal imbalances.

Avoiding certain negative lifestyle factors is essential. Alcohol consumption and smoking, for instance, have been linked to reduced testosterone levels and should be limited or avoided.

Rationale for Alternatives

Exploring the need for alternatives to testosterone therapy is driven by a growing recognition of the risks and side effects associated with hormonal treatments. Testosterone therapy, while beneficial for certain medical conditions, is not devoid of potential complications. These can range from mild side effects to more serious health risks, prompting both patients and healthcare providers to consider alternative methods for managing symptoms associated with low testosterone or hormonal imbalances.

One of the primary reasons for seeking alternatives is the risk of cardiovascular issues. Testosterone therapy has been linked in some studies to an increased risk of heart attacks and strokes, especially in older men or those with pre-existing heart conditions. Given the gravity of these potential outcomes, exploring safer options becomes a priority for many.

Another concern is the impact of testosterone therapy on prostate health. Testosterone can stimulate the growth of the prostate gland, and there is concern about its use in men with a history of prostate cancer, as it may accelerate the growth of cancer cells. Additionally, testosterone therapy can exacerbate symptoms of benign prostatic hyperplasia (BPH), leading to urinary problems.

The potential for endocrine system disruption is also a significant consideration. Long-term use of external testosterone can lead to a decrease in the body's natural hormone production, creating a dependency on the therapy. This can result in challenges when discontinuing the therapy, including withdrawal symptoms and a rebound effect.

Mental health side effects, such as mood swings, irritability, and increased aggression, are also notable concerns. Testosterone can significantly impact mood and behavior, and for some individuals, these changes can be detrimental, affecting their quality of life and interpersonal relationships.

There are also practical considerations, such as the inconvenience of ongoing therapy and the cost, which can be prohibitive for some individuals. Testosterone therapy often requires regular doctor visits, continuous monitoring, and lifelong treatment, which can be burdensome both in terms of time and finances.

Given these risks and challenges, the interest in alternatives to testosterone therapy is understandable. These alternatives range from lifestyle and dietary modifications to non-hormonal medications and natural supplements. Such approaches aim to address the underlying causes of low testosterone or manage its symptoms without the need for hormone replacement. For instance, regular exercise, particularly strength training, and a balanced diet can naturally boost testosterone levels. Stress reduction techniques can also play a role, as chronic stress is known to negatively affect hormone levels.

Exploring Alternative Treatments

Holistic and integrative medicine offers a broad spectrum of approaches to address conditions commonly treated with testosterone therapy, emphasizing the treatment of the whole person rather than focusing solely on hormone replacement. This field combines conventional medical practices with alternative therapies, creating a comprehensive, patient-centered approach to health and wellness. By exploring various methods under the umbrella of holistic and integrative medicine, patients and healthcare providers can address conditions such as low testosterone, aging-related hormonal changes, and associated symptoms in a more rounded and potentially less invasive manner.

One key aspect of holistic medicine is the focus on lifestyle modifications. Regular physical activity, particularly strength training and high-intensity interval exercises, has been shown to naturally boost testosterone levels. Additionally, practices such as yoga and Tai Chi not only improve physical strength and flexibility but also contribute to stress reduction, which can positively impact hormone levels. Sleep quality is another crucial factor; adequate, restful sleep plays a significant role in the regulation of hormones, including testosterone.

Dietary approaches are also integral to holistic and integrative medicine. Diets rich in certain nutrients can support the body's natural hormone production. Foods high in zinc (such as oysters, beef, and pumpkin seeds), magnesium (found in leafy greens, nuts, and whole grains), and omega-3 fatty acids (present in fatty fish and flaxseeds) can be beneficial. Conversely, reducing the intake of processed foods, sugars, and excessive carbohydrates can also positively affect hormone levels.

Herbal and natural supplements represent another approach within holistic medicine. While the efficacy of these supplements can vary, some, like fenugreek, ashwagandha, and ginger, have been studied for their potential to naturally support testosterone levels. However, it's important to approach supplements with caution, considering potential interactions with other medications and the variability in supplement quality.

Mind-body techniques are a cornerstone of integrative medicine, focusing on the connection between mental and physical health. Stress management techniques such as mindfulness meditation, deep breathing exercises, and biofeedback can be effective in reducing stress and anxiety, which in turn can positively influence hormonal balance.

Traditional medicine systems, such as Traditional Chinese Medicine (TCM) and Ayurveda, also offer perspectives and treatments that can be integrated into a holistic approach. These systems often utilize a combination of dietary advice, herbal remedies, and physical therapies like acupuncture to address hormonal imbalances and improve overall well-being.

In addition to these methods, integrative medicine also emphasizes the importance of addressing mental and emotional health. Counseling, cognitive-behavioral therapy, and other psychotherapeutic approaches can be instrumental in managing the psychological aspects associated with hormonal imbalances, such as mood swings, depression, and anxiety.

Finally, patient education and empowerment are key components of holistic and integrative medicine. Educating patients about the factors that influence hormonal health and involving them actively in their treatment decisions can lead to more successful outcomes.

Holistic and integrative medicine offers a diverse array of methods to address conditions treated with testosterone. By combining lifestyle changes, dietary modifications, herbal supplements, mind-body techniques, traditional medicine practices, and a focus on mental health, this approach provides a comprehensive framework for managing hormonal imbalances. It represents a patient-centered approach that not only addresses the physical aspects of health but also acknowledges the importance of mental and emotional well-being.

Patient Education

Patient education plays a pivotal role in the realm of healthcare, especially concerning treatments like testosterone therapy. The importance of informed decision-making cannot be overstated, as it empowers patients to actively participate in their healthcare journey, leading to better outcomes and higher satisfaction. In the context of hormone therapies, where potential risks and benefits need to be carefully weighed, being well-informed is crucial for patients to make choices that align with their health needs and personal values.

Firstly, patient education helps demystify medical information, making it more accessible and understandable. Medical treatments and their implications can often be complex and challenging to grasp. Effective patient education breaks down this complexity, presenting information in a clear, concise, and relevant manner. This is particularly important in the case of testosterone therapy, where patients must understand not only the potential benefits and improvements in symptoms but also the possible side effects and long-term health implications.

Informed decision-making also involves understanding the full spectrum of available options. For testosterone therapy, this means not only understanding the different types of treatments and methods of administration but also being aware of alternative and complementary therapies. Knowledge about lifestyle changes, dietary modifications, and other non-hormonal interventions offers patients a broader perspective, enabling them to make choices that are more aligned with their preferences and health goals.

Furthermore, patient education facilitates a more productive and collaborative patient-provider relationship. When patients are well-informed, they are better equipped to engage in meaningful conversations with their healthcare providers, ask pertinent questions, and express any concerns they might have. This two-way communication is essential for tailoring treatment plans to individual needs and for making adjustments as therapy progresses.

Another critical aspect of informed decision-making is the understanding of the risks associated with non-compliance or misuse of therapy. Education about the importance of adhering to the prescribed treatment regimen, the dangers of self-medication, and the potential for abuse underscores the seriousness of hormone therapy. It also highlights the importance of regular follow-ups and monitoring.

Patient education also includes preparing individuals for what to expect during therapy. This preparation can range from managing expectations regarding the onset and extent of benefits to recognizing and handling potential side effects. Being forewarned and forearmed helps patients to navigate their treatment journey more effectively and reduces anxiety or uncertainty about the process.

Informed decision-making is an ongoing process, not a one-time event. As patients progress through their treatment, their needs, and circumstances may change. Continuous education ensures that they remain well-informed throughout their therapy, enabling them to make decisions that are appropriate for their evolving health status.

Exercise and Physical Activity

Exercise and physical activity play a vital role in naturally boosting testosterone levels, offering a beneficial and non-invasive approach to managing hormonal health. Various forms of exercise have been shown to influence testosterone production, each in unique ways. Understanding how different types of physical activities impact testosterone levels can help individuals tailor their exercise routines to optimize hormonal health.

Strength training, or resistance training, is one of the most effective forms of exercise for increasing testosterone levels. Activities that involve lifting weights or using resistance bands lead to muscle growth and strength, which in turn stimulate the production of testosterone. Compound movements, such as squats, deadlifts, and bench presses, which work multiple muscle groups, are particularly effective. For optimal results, it's recommended to focus on heavier weights with fewer repetitions, as this has been shown to have a more significant impact on testosterone levels.

High-intensity interval training (HIIT) is another powerful way to boost testosterone. HIIT involves short bursts of intense activity followed by brief periods of rest or lower-intensity exercise. This type of training not only increases testosterone but also improves overall cardiovascular health and metabolism. HIIT can be applied to various forms of exercise, including running, cycling, rowing, or bodyweight exercises.

Aerobic exercises, such as running, swimming, or cycling, can also positively affect testosterone levels, particularly when performed at a moderate intensity. While the impact on testosterone might be less pronounced compared to strength training or HIIT, aerobic exercises contribute to overall health and help in maintaining a healthy weight, which is beneficial for hormonal balance.

Another aspect of physical activity that influences testosterone levels is consistency and variation in exercise routines. Regular physical activity is key to maintaining optimal testosterone levels, but it's also important to vary workouts to prevent plateauing effects. Incorporating a mix of strength training, HIIT, and aerobic exercises can provide a comprehensive workout regime that keeps the body challenged and hormones balanced.

It's also worth noting the importance of balance and recovery in an exercise routine. Overtraining or excessive exercise can lead to fatigue and stress, which may actually lower testosterone levels. Ensuring adequate rest, including good sleep quality and rest days in an exercise routine, is crucial for allowing the body to recover and maintain healthy hormone production.

In addition to exercise, other lifestyle factors such as diet, stress management, and overall health play a significant role in testosterone levels. A balanced approach that combines exercise with a healthy lifestyle is the most effective strategy for naturally managing testosterone levels.

Exercise and physical activity are powerful tools for naturally boosting testosterone levels. Strength training, high-intensity interval training, and aerobic exercises each contribute uniquely to hormonal health. Consistency, variation, balance, and recovery are key aspects of an exercise regime that aims to optimize testosterone levels. Integrating these forms of exercise with a healthy overall lifestyle can lead to significant improvements in hormonal balance and general well-being.

Diet and Nutrition

Diet and nutrition play a crucial role in influencing testosterone production, offering a natural and effective way to manage hormonal health. The relationship between what we eat and hormonal balance is significant, as certain foods and nutrients can either boost or hinder testosterone levels. Understanding this connection can help individuals make dietary choices that support their hormonal and overall health.

One of the key nutrients that influence testosterone production is zinc. Zinc is essential for the production of testosterone and other hormones. Foods rich in zinc include oysters (which have the highest concentration of zinc), red meat, poultry, beans, nuts, and whole grains. Including these foods in the diet can help maintain adequate zinc levels, which is crucial for testosterone production.

Vitamin D is another important nutrient for testosterone levels. It acts more like a hormone than a vitamin and has been shown to have a significant impact on testosterone production. Natural sources of vitamin D include fatty fish like salmon, mackerel, and sardines, fish liver oils, and egg yolks. Exposure to sunlight also stimulates the body to produce vitamin D, so spending time outdoors can boost levels naturally.

Healthy fats, particularly omega-3 fatty acids, are beneficial for hormonal health, including testosterone. These fats are essential for the production and regulation of hormones. Foods rich in omega-3s include flaxseeds, walnuts, and fatty fish like salmon and mackerel. Incorporating these into the diet can support healthy testosterone levels.

Magnesium is another mineral that plays a role in testosterone production. It helps to increase testosterone levels by reducing oxidative stress in the body. Foods high in magnesium include leafy green vegetables (such as spinach and Swiss chard), legumes, nuts, seeds, and whole grains.

Apart from specific nutrients, overall dietary patterns also impact testosterone levels. Diets that are high in processed foods, excessive sugars, and unhealthy fats can lead to obesity and insulin resistance, both of which are linked to lower testosterone levels. On the other hand, a balanced diet that includes a variety of whole foods, such as fruits, vegetables, whole grains, lean proteins, and healthy fats, can support hormonal health and overall well-being.

Reducing alcohol intake is also important for maintaining healthy testosterone levels. Excessive alcohol consumption can lead to a decrease in testosterone levels and negatively impact overall hormonal balance.

Hydration is another often-overlooked aspect of diet that can influence testosterone. Staying well-hydrated is essential for all aspects of health, including hormonal balance.

It's important to note that no single food or nutrient will drastically change testosterone levels on its own. A holistic approach to diet, focusing on overall nutrition and lifestyle, is the most effective way to support hormonal health.

Stress Reduction

Stress reduction is an essential aspect of managing hormone levels, including testosterone. The impact of stress on the body's hormonal balance is profound and multifaceted, with chronic stress being particularly detrimental to testosterone levels. Understanding the relationship between stress and hormones, and implementing effective strategies to manage stress, is crucial for maintaining hormonal health and overall well-being.

When the body is under stress, it produces higher levels of cortisol, a hormone released by the adrenal glands. Cortisol is known as the "stress hormone" because it helps the body respond to stress. However, when cortisol levels are consistently high due to chronic stress, it can lead to a hormonal imbalance. Elevated cortisol negatively impacts the production of testosterone, as the body prioritizes the production of stress-related hormones over other hormonal processes. This can result in lower testosterone levels, which can affect various aspects of health, including mood, libido, muscle mass, and energy levels.

Managing stress, therefore, becomes a key component in maintaining healthy testosterone levels. There are several effective methods to reduce stress:

- Mindfulness and Meditation: Practices like mindfulness and meditation can significantly reduce stress levels. These practices involve focusing on the present moment and becoming more aware of your thoughts and feelings without judgment. Regular meditation has been shown to decrease cortisol levels, thereby potentially improving testosterone levels.

- Exercise: Physical activity is a powerful stress reliever. Exercise not only improves physical health but also boosts endorphins, chemicals in the brain that are natural stress relievers. Exercise can also help mitigate some of the adverse effects of low testosterone, such as mood swings and fatigue.

- Adequate Sleep: Sleep is crucial for overall health and hormonal balance. Lack of sleep or poor-quality sleep can increase stress and disrupt hormone production, including testosterone. Ensuring 7-9 hours of quality sleep each night can help manage stress and support hormonal health.

- Yoga and Tai Chi: These ancient practices combine physical postures, breathing exercises, and meditation. They are particularly effective in reducing stress and have been shown to lower cortisol levels.

- Time Management: Effective time management can reduce the feeling of being overwhelmed, a common source of stress. Prioritizing tasks, setting realistic goals, and taking breaks can help manage workload and reduce stress.

- Social Support: Having a strong social network can help manage stress. Spending time with friends and family, or participating in group activities, can provide emotional support and alleviate stress.

- Relaxation Techniques: Techniques such as deep breathing exercises, progressive muscle relaxation, or listening to calming music can activate the body's relaxation response, counteracting the stress response.

- **Professional Help:** For chronic or severe stress, seeking help from a mental health professional can be beneficial. Therapy or counseling can provide strategies to manage stress effectively.

Managing stress is vital for maintaining healthy testosterone levels and overall well-being. Various techniques, including mindfulness, exercise, adequate sleep, yoga, effective time management, social support, relaxation techniques, and professional help, can be used to reduce stress. Incorporating these methods into daily life can help mitigate the negative impact of stress on hormonal balance, including testosterone levels.

Overview of Natural Supplements

Exploring the world of natural supplements provides a fascinating insight into how various herbs and natural substances can influence testosterone levels. The use of these supplements has been rooted in traditional medicine for centuries, and modern research is beginning to shed light on their potential effects and mechanisms. These natural agents offer a complementary approach to managing hormonal health, particularly for those seeking alternatives to conventional hormone therapies.

Among the myriad of natural supplements, certain herbs stand out for their potential impact on testosterone levels. One such herb is Fenugreek, a common ingredient in many cuisines, which has shown promise in some studies for its ability to boost testosterone. The mechanisms behind its effects are not entirely clear, but it's believed that compounds in fenugreek can stimulate the production of testosterone or enhance its release.

Another notable herb is Ashwagandha, an adaptogen revered in Ayurvedic medicine for its stress-reducing properties. Stress and hormone levels are intricately connected, and by reducing stress, ashwagandha may help improve the body's hormonal balance, including the regulation of testosterone. Clinical studies have suggested that ashwagandha not only reduces stress and anxiety but also boosts testosterone levels and improves sperm quality in men.

Tribulus terrestris is another supplement commonly associated with testosterone. Used in traditional Chinese and Indian medicine, it has been popular among athletes and bodybuilders. While some studies suggest it may improve sexual function and increase testosterone levels, the scientific evidence is mixed, and more research is needed to fully understand its effects.

Ginger, a widely used spice, also holds potential in influencing testosterone levels. Research has indicated that ginger supplementation can increase testosterone levels, with studies suggesting it may enhance luteinizing hormone production, a key hormone in regulating testosterone synthesis.

D-Aspartic Acid, an amino acid, is another supplement that has gained attention for its potential effects on testosterone. It plays a role in the production and release of testosterone, and some studies have shown that supplementation can temporarily boost low testosterone levels, particularly in men with impaired sexual function or fertility.

It's important to note, however, that while these natural supplements offer potential benefits, they are not without limitations. The effects of these supplements can vary greatly among individuals, and not all have been consistently backed by robust scientific evidence. Additionally, natural does not always mean safe; these supplements can interact with medications and may have side effects, especially when taken in high doses or for prolonged periods.

When considering natural supplements to influence testosterone levels, it's crucial to approach them as part of a broader health strategy. This strategy should include a balanced diet, regular exercise, stress management, and adequate sleep – all key factors in maintaining hormonal health. Consulting with healthcare professionals before starting any supplement regimen is also essential to ensure safety and appropriateness, especially for individuals with existing health conditions or those taking other medications.

Efficacy and Safety

The efficacy and safety of natural supplements as alternatives to conventional testosterone therapy are areas of growing interest and research. While there is a considerable body of anecdotal evidence supporting the use of various herbs and natural substances to influence testosterone levels, the scientific evidence varies in terms of robustness and consistency. A critical review of this evidence, alongside an understanding of the safety profiles of these alternatives, is essential for making informed decisions about their use.

Starting with Fenugreek, several studies have shown its potential in boosting testosterone levels and enhancing sexual function. The efficacy of fenugreek may stem from its compounds, such as furostanolic saponins, believed to stimulate testosterone production. However, while some clinical trials have reported positive results, others have shown minimal or no significant impact, indicating a need for further research to fully understand its effects.

Ashwagandha, known for its stress-reducing properties, has shown more consistent results in its ability to improve testosterone levels, particularly in stress-related scenarios. Clinical studies have demonstrated its effectiveness in enhancing sperm quality and increasing testosterone levels in men experiencing stress or fertility issues. This consistency makes ashwagandha a promising natural supplement for testosterone management.

Tribulus terrestris, popular among athletes for its supposed testosterone-boosting effects, has a more mixed scientific backing. Some studies have suggested improvements in sexual function and testosterone levels, particularly in men with sexual dysfunction. However, other research, including studies on healthy individuals, has not found significant changes in testosterone levels, casting doubt on its efficacy for broader use.

Ginger's impact on testosterone is supported by some studies, which have indicated that ginger supplementation can increase testosterone levels. These studies suggest that ginger may enhance luteinizing hormone production, important for testosterone synthesis. However, the research is still in its early stages, and more comprehensive studies are needed to confirm these findings.

D-Aspartic Acid has been shown to increase testosterone levels temporarily in certain groups, particularly those with low testosterone or impaired fertility. However, its effectiveness in healthy individuals or over the long term is less clear, with some studies showing no significant impact on testosterone levels.

In terms of safety, while these natural supplements are generally considered safe when used in moderation, they can have side effects and interact with other medications.

Fenugreek, for instance, can cause gastrointestinal discomfort and may interact with blood-thinning medications. Ashwagandha is usually well-tolerated but may cause drowsiness and should be used cautiously by those taking sedatives or thyroid medication. Tribulus terrestris is also generally safe but can cause stomach issues and should be avoided by those with hormone-sensitive conditions like prostate cancer. Ginger is widely regarded as safe but can interact with blood thinners and diabetes medications. D-Aspartic Acid is generally safe but can cause gastrointestinal side effects and irritability in some individuals.

It's crucial to approach these supplements with a comprehensive understanding of both their potential benefits and limitations. The variation in study results and potential side effects underscores the importance of personalized healthcare and the need for more research. Anyone considering natural supplements for testosterone management should consult with a healthcare professional to ensure that their choice aligns with their overall health profile and treatment goals.

While natural supplements like fenugreek, ashwagandha, Tribulus terrestris, ginger, and D-Aspartic Acid show promise in influencing testosterone levels, the scientific evidence supporting their efficacy is varied. Considering their safety profiles and potential interactions, these supplements should be used judiciously and under the guidance of a healthcare professional. This approach ensures that individuals can safely explore natural alternatives as part of a holistic strategy for managing hormonal health.

Non-Hormonal Pharmaceutical Options

Exploring non-hormonal pharmaceutical options presents a significant avenue for individuals seeking alternatives to traditional testosterone therapy. These medications offer potential benefits for managing symptoms associated with low testosterone or hormonal imbalances without directly altering hormone levels. This approach can be particularly appealing for those who are either unable to use hormone therapy due to medical reasons or who prefer to avoid the potential side effects associated with hormonal treatments.

One category of non-hormonal medications that has garnered attention is selective estrogen receptor modulators (SERMs). These drugs, typically used in treating breast cancer and osteoporosis, can also impact testosterone levels indirectly. By modulating estrogen receptors, SERMs can lead to a decrease in estrogen levels and an increase in the body's natural production of testosterone. However, their use for this purpose is off-label, and more research is needed to fully understand their efficacy and safety in managing low testosterone.

Another class of drugs worth noting is aromatase inhibitors. Aromatase is an enzyme that converts testosterone into estrogen. Aromatase inhibitors, therefore, can help increase testosterone levels by preventing this conversion. These medications are often used in the treatment of breast cancer but have also been explored for managing conditions associated with low testosterone. However, their long-term effects and safety profile require careful consideration, especially since they can lead to reduced estrogen levels, which have their own health implications.

Phosphodiesterase type 5 (PDE5) inhibitors are commonly known for treating erectile dysfunction, a common symptom associated with low testosterone. While these drugs do not directly influence testosterone levels, they can improve sexual function, which is often affected in conditions of low testosterone. Medications like sildenafil (Viagra) and tadalafil (Cialis) fall into this category.

There are also medications that address specific symptoms associated with low testosterone, such as antidepressants for mood swings or medications for osteoporosis. These treatments can be particularly useful for managing individual symptoms without the broad systemic effects of testosterone therapy.

It's important to note that while these non-hormonal pharmaceutical options can offer benefits, they are not without risks and side effects. SERMs and aromatase inhibitors can cause joint pain, mood swings, and vision changes, among other side effects. PDE5 inhibitors can lead to headaches, flushing, and in rare cases, more serious cardiovascular events. As with any medication, the potential benefits must be weighed against the risks.

In addition, these medications often require careful monitoring and regular follow-ups with healthcare providers. This monitoring ensures that any adverse effects are quickly identified and managed, and that the medication's efficacy is evaluated over time.

Physical Therapies

Investigating physical therapies such as acupuncture or chiropractic care reveals an intriguing dimension in the management of conditions often treated with testosterone therapy. These physical treatments offer a non-pharmaceutical approach, focusing on the body's natural mechanisms to improve health and alleviate symptoms. While these therapies do not directly influence testosterone levels, they can be effective in managing certain symptoms associated with hormonal imbalances and contribute to overall well-being.

Acupuncture, a key component of traditional Chinese medicine, involves the insertion of fine needles into specific points on the body. This process is believed to stimulate the body's natural healing processes and balance the flow of energy, or Qi. In the context of hormonal health, acupuncture has been explored for its potential in alleviating symptoms such as stress, anxiety, and mood swings, which can be associated with hormonal imbalances. Some studies suggest that acupuncture can also improve sexual function and potentially impact hormone levels indirectly by reducing stress and improving overall health. However, the evidence is mixed, and more research is needed to fully understand its effects on hormonal conditions.

Chiropractic care, focusing on the diagnosis and treatment of musculoskeletal disorders, primarily through manual adjustment or manipulation of the spine, also holds potential benefits. While chiropractic treatments do not directly target hormonal imbalances, they can alleviate some of the symptoms associated with low testosterone, such as chronic pain, fatigue, and mood issues. By improving spinal alignment, chiropractic care may enhance the nervous system's function, leading to overall improved health and potentially impacting hormonal regulation indirectly.

In addition to these, other physical therapies such as massage therapy and osteopathy can contribute to overall health and wellness. Massage therapy can reduce stress and improve circulation, which might indirectly support better hormonal balance. Osteopathy, which involves the manipulation of the body's muscles and bones, can improve the body's mechanical function and alleviate stress, contributing to overall hormonal health.

It's important to approach these physical therapies as complementary treatments. They are most effective when used in conjunction with traditional medical treatments and lifestyle modifications. For individuals with conditions treated by testosterone therapy, these physical therapies can provide additional support, helping to manage symptoms and improve quality of life.

Safety and proper practice are crucial when considering physical therapies. Acupuncture should be performed by a licensed and experienced practitioner to ensure safety and effectiveness. Similarly, chiropractic care and other physical therapies should be conducted by qualified professionals to minimize any risks and maximize therapeutic benefits.

Psychological Counseling

The role of psychological counseling in managing symptoms associated with hormonal imbalances, particularly those related to testosterone levels, is a vital component of a comprehensive treatment plan. Mental health support through counseling offers a means to address the psychological and emotional aspects that often accompany hormonal disorders. This approach recognizes that the effects of hormonal imbalances are not just physical but also profoundly impact mental and emotional well-being.

Testosterone plays a significant role in mood regulation, energy levels, and overall mental health. Fluctuations or deficiencies in testosterone can lead to symptoms such as depression, anxiety, mood swings, and irritability. These psychological symptoms can be just as debilitating as the physical ones and require appropriate intervention. Psychological counseling provides a space for individuals to explore and understand these mental health challenges, offering strategies to cope with and manage them effectively.

Counseling can take various forms, including individual therapy, group therapy, or family/couples therapy, depending on the individual's needs and the nature of the symptoms. Cognitive-behavioral therapy (CBT) is particularly effective for managing depression and anxiety. It helps individuals recognize and change negative thought patterns and behaviors that contribute to their mental health challenges.

One of the key benefits of psychological counseling is the development of coping strategies. Individuals learn to manage stress, handle emotional ups and downs, and navigate the challenges that come with hormonal imbalances. Counseling can also provide support for related issues such as changes in sexual function or self-esteem, which are common concerns in those experiencing hormonal shifts.

Additionally, counseling offers a holistic approach to treatment. It recognizes the interconnectedness of physical and mental health, emphasizing the importance of addressing both aspects to achieve overall well-being. This approach can be particularly beneficial for individuals who are undergoing or considering hormone therapy, as it helps them to prepare mentally and emotionally for the treatment and its potential impacts.

In cases where hormonal imbalances affect interpersonal relationships, counseling can be invaluable. It can offer tools and techniques for communication and understanding, helping to mitigate the strain that these imbalances can place on relationships, whether they be romantic, familial, or professional.

It's also worth noting that psychological counseling can be beneficial not just for those directly experiencing hormonal issues, but also for their partners or family members. It provides education and understanding for loved ones, helping them to support the individual effectively.

Mind-Body Techniques

The role of mind-body techniques, particularly yoga, meditation, and mindfulness, in managing health and well-being has gained significant recognition in recent times. These practices offer a holistic approach to health, emphasizing the connection between the mind and body. In the context of managing symptoms associated with hormonal imbalances, such as those related to testosterone levels, these techniques can be particularly beneficial, providing a natural and non-invasive way to enhance overall health and mitigate symptoms.

Yoga, an ancient practice that combines physical postures, breathing exercises, and meditation, offers numerous health benefits. For individuals experiencing hormonal imbalances, yoga can be especially helpful. The physical postures (asanas) help improve strength and flexibility, which can boost physical well-being and body confidence. The breathing techniques (pranayama) used in yoga are effective in reducing stress and anxiety, factors that can influence hormonal balance. Furthermore, yoga has been shown to improve mood and mental clarity, helping to alleviate symptoms like depression and mood swings associated with low testosterone.

Meditation, a practice that involves focusing the mind and achieving a mentally clear and emotionally calm state, plays a significant role in stress reduction. Chronic stress is known to negatively impact hormone levels, including testosterone. Meditation can help lower stress hormones like cortisol, thereby potentially improving the hormonal balance in the body. Regular meditation practice has also been associated with improvements in sleep quality, another crucial factor in maintaining healthy hormone levels.

Mindfulness, a practice of being fully present and engaged in the moment without judgment, is another effective mind-body technique. Mindfulness can be practiced in various forms, including through mindfulness meditation, mindful eating, or simply incorporating mindfulness into daily activities. This practice helps individuals become more aware of their thoughts and feelings and teaches them to respond to stressors more calmly and effectively. By reducing stress and improving emotional well-being, mindfulness can indirectly support hormonal health.

These mind-body techniques not only address the physical and psychological symptoms associated with hormonal imbalances but also contribute to an overall sense of well-being. They encourage a deeper connection with the body, enhance self-awareness, and promote relaxation, all of which are beneficial in managing hormonal health.

It's important to note that while yoga, meditation, and mindfulness are powerful tools, they are most effective when used as part of a broader health management strategy. This strategy may include traditional medical treatments, lifestyle changes, and dietary modifications. Additionally, these mind-body techniques can be adapted to suit individual needs and abilities, making them accessible to a wide range of individuals.

Traditional Medicine Practices

The insights from traditional medicine practices such as Ayurveda and Traditional Chinese Medicine (TCM) offer a rich and diverse perspective on managing health, including hormonal imbalances. These ancient healing systems, with their holistic approach, provide a unique lens through which we can view and address conditions typically treated with testosterone therapy.

Ayurveda, an ancient Indian system of medicine, places great emphasis on balance in bodily systems using diet, herbal treatment, and yogic breathing. In Ayurveda, hormonal imbalances are often viewed through the lens of an imbalance in the body's fundamental energies, known as doshas. Treatments in Ayurveda for hormonal issues might include dietary changes, herbal remedies, and specific physical practices. For example, herbs like Ashwagandha are used for their adaptogenic properties, believed to support the body's stress response and potentially impact hormone levels. Ayurveda also emphasizes the importance of a balanced diet that supports the individual's dosha type, and practices like yoga and meditation for overall well-being.

Traditional Chinese Medicine, with its centuries-old history, offers another holistic approach. TCM views the body as a system of energy flows and balances. Treatment for hormonal imbalances often involves acupuncture, herbal medicine, and Qi Gong exercises. In

TCM, the goal is to restore balance and ensure the smooth flow of Qi (energy) throughout the body. Acupuncture, in particular, is used to target specific meridians or pathways to alleviate symptoms and restore balance. Herbs in TCM, like Ginseng, are often used for their supposed ability to support energy levels and improve vitality, which can be linked to hormonal health.

Both these systems also stress the importance of a harmonious lifestyle that aligns with natural rhythms and individual constitution. Practices such as proper sleep, stress management, and a diet suited to one's unique body type and environmental factors are considered crucial in maintaining hormonal balance.

It's important to recognize that while these traditional systems offer valuable insights and approaches, they are based on concepts and philosophies that differ from Western medicine. The efficacy of many of these practices and treatments has been supported by anecdotal evidence and some modern research, but more scientific studies are needed to fully understand their impact, particularly on hormonal health.

Furthermore, integrating traditional medicine practices with modern healthcare requires a thoughtful and informed approach. Individuals interested in exploring these avenues should consult with qualified practitioners who have expertise in these specific traditions. It's also crucial to communicate with healthcare providers about all aspects of an individual's treatment plan, including the use of traditional medicine practices, to ensure safe and coordinated care

How to Choose the Right Path

Choosing the right path in therapy, especially when it involves managing conditions like hormonal imbalances, requires a nuanced and individualized approach. The most appropriate therapy for an individual depends on a variety of factors including their specific symptoms, overall health, lifestyle, and personal preferences. Navigating this decision-making process involves careful consideration and often collaboration between the individual, healthcare providers, and possibly other wellness practitioners.

The first step in selecting the most appropriate therapy is a thorough medical evaluation. This should include a comprehensive assessment of symptoms, medical history, and current health status. Blood tests to measure hormone levels and other relevant markers can provide valuable insights into the individual's specific condition and needs. It's crucial that this evaluation is carried out by a qualified healthcare professional who can accurately interpret the results and recommend appropriate treatment options.

Understanding the individual's unique symptoms and how they impact their daily life is key to choosing the right therapy. For instance, if low testosterone is leading to severe fatigue that affects daily functioning, the treatment approach may differ from a situation where the primary concern is mild mood swings. The severity and impact of symptoms play a critical role in determining the most effective and appropriate treatment.

Lifestyle factors and overall health must also be taken into account. This includes considering the individual's age, dietary habits, physical activity levels, stress levels, and other health conditions they may have. For example, someone with a sedentary lifestyle and poor dietary habits might benefit significantly from lifestyle interventions alongside or even before considering medical therapies.

Patient preference and values are crucial in the decision-making process. Some individuals may prefer to explore natural or alternative therapies before considering hormone therapy, while others might prioritize a more immediate medical intervention. Understanding and respecting these preferences is vital for ensuring that the chosen therapy aligns with the individual's values and expectations.

It's also important to consider the potential risks and benefits of different therapies. Hormone therapy, for instance, can be very effective but also comes with potential side effects and risks. Non-hormonal options or lifestyle changes might offer a safer alternative but may take longer to produce results. A frank discussion with healthcare providers about the pros and cons of different treatment options is essential.

In cases where the chosen path involves complementary or alternative therapies, it's important to seek out qualified practitioners and ensure that these therapies do not conflict with any other ongoing treatments. Integrating different modalities of treatment should be done under the guidance of knowledgeable professionals.

Ongoing monitoring and adjustment are part of choosing the right therapy. What works initially may need to be adjusted over time as the individual's needs or health status change. Regular follow-ups with healthcare providers are crucial for monitoring the effectiveness of the therapy and making necessary adjustments.

Working with Healthcare Providers

Effective communication and collaboration with healthcare providers are fundamental for achieving the best health outcomes, especially when managing complex conditions like hormonal imbalances. Navigating the healthcare system and building a productive relationship with medical professionals require proactive and informed engagement from patients. Here are some tips for fostering effective communication and collaboration with healthcare providers.

Firstly, it's crucial to be prepared for medical appointments. This means gathering all relevant health information, including any symptoms you're experiencing, your medical history, current medications, and any supplements or alternative therapies you're using. Keeping a health diary can be particularly helpful, as it allows you to provide detailed information about your symptoms and how they affect your daily life.

Clear and honest communication is key. Be open about your symptoms, concerns, and any other health-related issues you're experiencing. Don't hesitate to ask questions about your condition, treatment options, potential side effects, and anything else you're uncertain about. If there's something you don't understand, ask for clarification. Remember, there are no silly questions when it comes to your health.

Active listening is just as important as sharing your concerns. Pay close attention to the information your healthcare provider gives you, and take notes if necessary. This can help you remember their advice and instructions after the appointment.

It's also beneficial to discuss your preferences and treatment goals with your healthcare provider. Whether you have a preference for certain types of treatments or specific concerns about side effects, sharing these with your provider can help them tailor your treatment plan to better suit your needs and expectations.

If you're considering alternative therapies or lifestyle changes, discuss these with your healthcare provider. They can provide valuable insights on how these might interact with your current treatment plan and overall health.

In cases where you're not fully satisfied with the information or treatment plan provided, don't hesitate to seek a second opinion. A different perspective can sometimes offer additional insights or alternative approaches to your treatment.

Collaborating with healthcare providers also means adhering to the agreed-upon treatment plan and following their recommendations. However, if you're facing challenges with the treatment, such as side effects or difficulties with adherence, communicate these issues during your follow-up appointments.

Building a long-term relationship with your healthcare provider is beneficial. When your provider is familiar with your health history and personal circumstances, they are better positioned to offer personalized care.

Emerging Therapies

The landscape of medical treatments is continually evolving, with emerging therapies offering new hope and options for managing various health conditions. In the realm of hormonal imbalances and conditions traditionally treated with testosterone therapy, several new and upcoming treatments show promise. These emerging therapies reflect advancements in medical research and technology, offering more targeted, efficient, and sometimes less invasive treatment options.

One of the exciting areas of development is in the field of gene therapy. Researchers are exploring the potential of gene therapy to directly influence hormone levels, including testosterone. This approach involves altering specific genes or gene expressions to correct hormonal imbalances at a molecular level. While still in the early stages of research, gene therapy could offer a more permanent solution to hormonal disorders, moving beyond managing symptoms to potentially addressing the root causes.

Another area of interest is peptide therapy, which involves using specific peptides to influence the body's hormonal functions. Peptides are short chains of amino acids that can act as signaling molecules in the body. By using peptides that mimic or influence hormones, researchers are exploring ways to naturally stimulate the body's hormone production or regulate hormonal activity. This approach could provide a more natural and less invasive alternative to traditional hormone replacement therapies.

Advancements in bioidentical hormone replacement therapy (BHRT) are also noteworthy. BHRT involves the use of hormones that are chemically identical to those the body produces naturally. Recent developments in BHRT include more precise dosing methods and delivery systems, such as transdermal patches or creams that provide a steady release of hormones, reducing the risk of fluctuations and side effects.

Nanotechnology is another frontier in the development of new treatments. Nanoparticles can be used to deliver medications more effectively to specific areas of the body. In the context of hormone therapy, this could mean more targeted delivery of hormone treatments with fewer systemic side effects.

Additionally, there is ongoing research into natural treatments and supplements, with a focus on identifying and validating the efficacy of various herbs, vitamins, and minerals in managing hormonal imbalances. This research is particularly important for individuals seeking natural or complementary alternatives to traditional medical treatments.

It's important to note that while these emerging therapies offer exciting prospects, they are often still in the experimental or testing phases. Clinical trials and rigorous scientific research are essential to establish their efficacy and safety before they become widely available as standard treatments.

The Importance of Research

The importance of research in the field of hormonal health and therapy cannot be overstated, as it is the cornerstone upon which effective and safe treatments are built. Continued scientific exploration in this area is essential for several compelling reasons.

Firstly, the complexity of the endocrine system and its profound impact on the human body necessitates a deep and evolving understanding. Hormones like testosterone play multifaceted roles, influencing not just physical aspects such as muscle mass and bone density, but also mental health, emotional well-being, and overall quality of life. Research helps unravel these complex interactions and effects, leading to more effective treatment strategies.

Advancements in technology and medical science open new avenues for treatments that need to be thoroughly explored and understood. Emerging therapies such as gene therapy, peptide therapy, and advanced forms of hormone replacement therapy hold great promise, but they also require rigorous scientific investigation to establish their efficacy, safety, and long-term effects. Research in these areas can lead to breakthroughs that offer more personalized, efficient, and less invasive treatment options.

Additionally, the variability in individual responses to hormone therapy underscores the need for personalized medicine. Research helps identify genetic, environmental, and lifestyle factors that influence these responses, allowing for more tailored and effective treatment plans. Understanding individual differences is crucial in optimizing treatment efficacy and minimizing side effects.

Ongoing research is also vital in addressing the challenges and risks associated with hormone therapy. For instance, studies exploring the long-term effects of testosterone therapy on cardiovascular health, prostate cancer risk, and mental health are critical for ensuring patient safety. This research can lead to improved guidelines and protocols that enhance the safety and effectiveness of hormone treatments.

Furthermore, the exploration of natural and alternative therapies for managing hormonal imbalances is an area ripe for research. While traditional and natural remedies are often used, scientific validation of their efficacy and safety is necessary for their integration into mainstream medicine. This research can provide individuals with more options and support a holistic approach to health care.

Research in hormonal health also has broader implications for public health. Hormonal imbalances are associated with various health conditions and diseases. Understanding these connections can lead to better prevention strategies, early detection methods, and more effective treatments, benefiting public health as a whole.

Research in this field is not just about developing new treatments but also about improving patient education and healthcare delivery. Studies focusing on the best ways to communicate complex medical information, engage patients in their treatment plans, and deliver care more effectively are essential for enhancing patient outcomes and satisfaction.

Key Takeaways

The exploration of testosterone therapy and its alternatives in this comprehensive guide traversed a broad spectrum of topics, providing a deep dive into the complexities of hormonal health and treatment. We began with an overview of testosterone therapy, defining it and discussing its common uses, especially in treating conditions like hypogonadism and addressing age-related testosterone decline. Delving into the historical background, we explored the evolution of testosterone use in medical practices, tracing its journey from early discoveries to the current trends in prescriptions. This historical perspective highlighted how perceptions and applications of testosterone therapy have changed over time.

We then delved into understanding testosterone in the human body, examining its biological roles in both males and females. This included a discussion on the natural fluctuations of testosterone levels and their implications, as well as the misconceptions surrounding the benefits of artificially elevated testosterone levels. The next section focused on the rise of testosterone therapy, particularly the influence of media and marketing. This analysis included how the media portrays testosterone therapy and the role of pharmaceutical marketing in promoting its use, supplemented by case studies of misleading or exaggerated advertising campaigns.

The book then transitioned to discussing the short-term and long-term side effects of testosterone therapy. Immediate physiological responses and common side effects experienced soon after therapy begins were covered, along with the psychological impacts such as mood swings and mental health concerns. Real-life examples and case studies provided a grounded understanding of these effects. Long-term health risks were also thoroughly examined, including the potential hormonal imbalance, cardiovascular risks, and disruption to the endocrine system. Specific risks by demographic, like age-related risks and gender-specific concerns, were discussed in detail, emphasizing the varying effects of testosterone therapy across different groups.

The psychological and behavioral effects of testosterone therapy were another key focus, exploring how the therapy can lead to mental health risks and behavioral changes such as increased aggression and risk-taking behavior. The societal and ethical implications were then scrutinized, delving into the social pressures and body image issues associated with testosterone therapy and the ethical responsibilities of healthcare providers in prescribing and managing therapy.

Regulatory and ethical considerations were explored, providing an overview of the regulatory landscape governing testosterone prescriptions and the ethical considerations in prescribing testosterone, especially in vulnerable populations. Recommendations for policy changes and improved regulatory oversight were proposed to enhance patient safety and the effectiveness of treatments.

Looking towards the future, the book highlighted emerging research and future directions in hormone therapy, discussing the potential for more precise and safer treatments. Guidelines for navigating testosterone therapy safely were provided, covering best practices for safe use, monitoring and managing side effects, and understanding when testosterone therapy might not be the right choice.

Alternative approaches and preventative measures were extensively covered, including natural testosterone management, the rationale for alternatives due to risks and side effects associated with testosterone therapy, and holistic and integrative medicine practices. The importance of lifestyle and dietary modifications was underscored, as well as the role of herbal and natural supplements. Non-hormonal medical interventions, integrative and holistic approaches, and navigating treatment options were also discussed.

Finally, the book concluded by emphasizing the importance of making empowering choices and encouraging a cautious and informed approach to testosterone therapy. Appendices provided additional resources, including a glossary of medical terms and resources for further information, rounding out a comprehensive guide to understanding and managing testosterone therapy and its alternatives.

Empowering Choices

In the journey through the intricacies of testosterone therapy and its alternatives, the overarching theme has been one of empowering choices, encouraging readers to make informed decisions about their health and wellness. The detailed exploration of this subject, from the historical context to the current trends, and from the biological implications to the societal impact, is aimed at providing a comprehensive understanding that equips individuals with the knowledge needed to navigate their health choices effectively.

This empowerment begins with a clear comprehension of the role and effects of testosterone in the body, both in its natural state and when supplemented through therapy. Understanding the balance required in the body's hormonal system is crucial, as is recognizing the potential risks and benefits of altering this balance. The exploration of short-term and long-term side effects, along with the demographic-specific risks, serves to highlight the importance of considering personal health circumstances and needs when contemplating testosterone therapy.

Psychological and behavioral aspects form a crucial part of this decision-making process. Acknowledging and understanding the potential mental and emotional impacts of testosterone therapy are vital. Similarly, being aware of societal pressures and ethical considerations surrounding testosterone use adds another layer to the informed decision-making process.

The regulatory landscape and the ethical responsibilities of healthcare providers have been detailed not just for academic understanding but to empower readers in their interactions with healthcare professionals. This knowledge facilitates more meaningful discussions with healthcare providers, ensuring that treatment decisions are collaborative, well-informed, and personalized.

Additionally, the book delves into various alternatives to traditional testosterone therapy, including lifestyle and dietary modifications, herbal supplements, and non-hormonal medical interventions. These alternatives provide options for those seeking different approaches, reflecting the diverse needs and preferences of individuals. Understanding these alternatives widens the spectrum of choices available, enabling readers to consider a range of strategies in managing their health.

Emerging therapies and future directions in hormone therapy research have been highlighted to give readers insights into what the future holds in this field. This forward-looking perspective ensures that readers are not only informed about current practices but are also aware of potential future developments.

Glossary of Terms

Here are some key terms that are essential for understanding the content discussed in the book:

- Androgen: A type of hormone that plays a role in male traits and reproductive activity; testosterone is a primary androgen.

- Aromatase Inhibitors: Medications that stop the conversion of androgens into estrogen, used in the treatment of breast cancer and conditions involving estrogen-sensitive tissues.

- Bioidentical Hormones: Hormones that are chemically identical to those the human body produces; often used in hormone replacement therapy.

- Endocrine System: The network of glands in the body that produce hormones, which regulate many of the body's functions including growth, metabolism, and sexual function.

- Erectile Dysfunction: The inability to get or keep an erection firm enough for sexual intercourse, often associated with low testosterone levels.

- Gonadotropin-releasing Hormone (GnRH): A hormone produced in the hypothalamus that signals the pituitary gland to release gonadotropins, which in turn stimulate the gonads to produce sex hormones.

- Hypogonadism: A condition in which the body doesn't produce enough testosterone.

- Luteinizing Hormone (LH): A hormone produced by the pituitary gland that plays a key role in controlling the function of the testes in men and ovaries in women.

- Phosphodiesterase type 5 (PDE5) Inhibitors: A class of drugs that inhibit the enzyme PDE5, used to treat erectile dysfunction and some other conditions.

- Polycythemia: An increased number of red blood cells in the blood, which can be a side effect of testosterone therapy.

- Selective Estrogen Receptor Modulators (SERMs): Drugs that act on the estrogen receptor, used in the treatment of breast cancer and osteoporosis, and investigated for their effects on testosterone levels.

- Testosterone: The primary male sex hormone responsible for the development of male reproductive tissues and the promotion of secondary sexual characteristics.

- Testosterone Therapy: Medical treatment intended to boost levels of testosterone in individuals where it is low due to medical conditions.

- Tribulus Terrestris: A plant used in traditional medicine, often claimed to improve sexual function and increase testosterone levels.

Understanding these terms is crucial for a comprehensive grasp of the discussions on hormonal health, therapies, and treatments. This glossary serves as a quick reference to demystify medical jargon and enhance the reader's understanding of the subject matter.

Resources

The following resources offer reliable and comprehensive information that can enhance understanding and provide additional support:

- Endocrine Society: A leading organization in the field of endocrinology, offering a wealth of resources on hormonal health, including patient-focused information on testosterone therapy. Their website (www.endocrine.org) features educational materials, clinical guidelines, and the latest research findings.

- American Urological Association: Provides resources and information related to men's health, including testosterone therapy and hormonal imbalances (www.auanet.org). They offer patient guides, clinical guidelines, and updates on recent research.

- National Institute on Aging: Offers information on health issues related to aging, including hormonal changes (www.nia.nih.gov). This resource is valuable for understanding age-related hormonal decline and management strategies.

- Mayo Clinic: A renowned medical center offering extensive patient education materials on a wide range of health topics, including testosterone and hormonal health (www.mayoclinic.org). Their website provides detailed articles, symptom checkers, and treatment options.

- PubMed: A database of scientific studies and reviews (www.pubmed.gov). For those interested in delving into the research literature on testosterone therapy and hormonal health, PubMed offers access to a vast array of academic and clinical studies.

- Men's Health Network: An organization dedicated to men's health, providing education, screenings, and advocacy (www.menshealthnetwork.org). They offer resources specific to men's hormonal health and wellness.

- Women's Health Research Institute: Offers resources and information on women's health, including hormonal balance (www.womenshealthresearch.org). While testosterone is often associated with men's health, it plays a significant role in women's health as well.

- Books and Academic Journals: Reading books written by experts in the field, as well as academic journals like "The Journal of Clinical Endocrinology & Metabolism" and "The Journal of Men's Health," can provide in-depth insights and the latest research findings.

- Online Support Groups and Forums: Platforms like HealthUnlocked (www.healthunlocked.com) offer online communities where individuals can share experiences and advice on managing hormonal health.

- Your Healthcare Provider: Always a primary and essential resource. For personalized medical advice, diagnosis, or treatment, consulting with healthcare professionals is crucial.

These resources provide a starting point for further exploration into the subject of testosterone therapy and hormonal health. They offer a range of perspectives from patient education to scientific research, aiding in a well-rounded understanding of these complex topics.

Disclaimer

The content of this book, including but not limited to text, graphics, images, and other material, is for informational purposes only and is not intended to be a substitute for professional medical advice, diagnosis, or treatment. The information provided in this book should not be used for diagnosing or treating a health problem or disease, or prescribing any medication or other treatment.

Always seek the advice of your physician or other qualified health provider with any questions you may have regarding a medical condition. Never disregard professional medical advice or delay in seeking it because of something you have read in this book. The authors and publishers of this book do not assume any liability for the information contained herein, be it direct, indirect, consequential, special, exemplary, or other damages.

The views expressed in this book are those of the authors and do not necessarily reflect the official policy or position of any medical or health organization. Reliance on any information provided in this book is solely at your own risk. The mention of specific products, processes, or services in this book does not constitute or imply a recommendation or endorsement by the authors or publishers.